With over 40 million Americ
carbohydrate intake, the n
formation and counters. N
figures—those that relate .
one groundbreaking reference that will redefine the way you
eat carbs forever.

THE ESSENTIAL NET CARB COUNTER

A "net carb" refers to a carbohydrate that is digested by the body but not turned into glucose, or a carbohydrate that is not digested at all. These types of carbohydrates are "safe" and do not negatively impact weight loss. Here, for the first time, nutrition expert Maggie Robinson, Ph.D., provides a comprehensive book of "net carb" listings, while also providing straight-up carb counts, and calorie and fiber counts.

THE ESSENTIAL NET CARB COUNTER

Maggie Greenwood-Robinson, Ph.D.

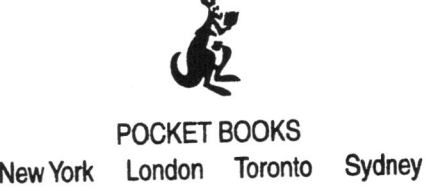

POCKET BOOKS
New York   London   Toronto   Sydney

The sale of this book without its cover is unauthorized. If you purchased this book without a cover, you should be aware that it was reported to the publisher as "unsold and destroyed." Neither the author nor the publisher has received payment for the sale of this "stripped book."

An *Original* Publication of POCKET BOOKS

 POCKET BOOKS, a division of Simon & Schuster, Inc.
1230 Avenue of the Americas, New York, NY 10020

Copyright © 2005 by Maggie Greenwood-Robinson, Ph.D.

All rights reserved, including the right to reproduce this book or portions thereof in any form whatsoever. For information address Pocket Books, 1230 Avenue of the Americas, New York, NY 10020

ISBN: 978-1-4767-9120-3

First Pocket Books printing January 2005

10 9 8 7 6 5

POCKET and colophon are registered trademarks of Simon & Schuster, Inc.

Cover art by Anna Dorfman

Manufactured in the United States of America

For information regarding special discounts for bulk purchases, please contact Simon & Schuster Special Sales at 1-800-456-6798 or business@simonandschuster.com.

Every effort has been made to ensure that the information contained in this book is complete and accurate. However, neither the publisher nor the author is engaged in rendering professional advice or services to the individual reader. The ideas, procedures, and suggestions contained in this book are not intended as a substitute for consulting with your physician. All matters regarding your health require medical supervision. Neither the author nor the publisher shall be liable or responsible for any loss, injury, or damage allegedly arising from any information or suggestions in this book. The opinions expressed in this book represent the personal views of the author and not of the publisher.

ACKNOWLEDGMENTS

There are always many people to thank for the opportunity to write a book, and therefore I would like to thank Micki Nuding and the staff at Pocket Books for their innovative thinking that a book like this is needed at this time. Appreciation also goes to my agent Madeleine Morel, with whom I have worked for many, many years, and whose guidance has been invaluable.

Most of all, I would like to thank the principal researcher for this book, Jeff Robinson, NSCA-CPT, who is one of the best fitness experts and trainers in the United States today.

CONTENTS

Foreword by Robert Monaco, M.D., M.P.H. — xi
Introduction: Let the Net Carb Countdown Begin! — 1

The Essential Net Carb Counter

- Alcoholic Beverages — 17
- Bagels and Bread Products — 21
- Beans and Legumes — 29
- Beef — 31
- Bread — 40
- Cake — 43
- Candy — 47
- Cereals — 65
- Cheese — 75
- Coffee and Tea — 77
- Condiments and Mayonnaise — 80
- Cookies and Brownies — 83
- Cream and Creamers — 94
- Diet and Nutritional Bars, Cereal Bars — 95
- Dips and Spreads — 107
- Eggs — 109
- Entrées — 109
- Fast Food and Other Restaurants — 120
- Fats and Oils — 219
- Fish and Shellfish — 227
- Frostings and Toppings — 234
- Fruits and Fruit Juices — 236
- Game Meats, Lean — 249

CONTENTS

Grains and Grain Cakes	250
Hot Dogs	251
Ice Cream and Frozen Desserts	251
Ice Cream Bars and Pops	256
Jam, Sugar, Syrup, and Sweeteners	257
Lamb	266
Lunch Meats	268
Milk and Milk Beverages	270
Nutritional Drinks and Shakes	272
Nuts, Nut Butters, and Seeds	278
Organ Meats	281
Pancakes and Waffles	281
Pasta and Noodles	284
Pastries and Donuts	288
Pickles and Olives	293
Pies and Pie Fillings	294
Pizzas	297
Pork, Ham, and Bacon	300
Pork Products	301
Poultry	302
Puddings	306
Salad Dressings	308
Sauces, Gravies, and Marinades	311
Sausage, Lean	317
Snack Foods (Chips, Crackers, Popcorn, Pretzels, and Others)	317
Soft Drinks	330
Soups	332
Soy and Vegetarian Foods	342
Veal	343
Vegetables and Vegetable Juices	345
Yogurt	368

Appendix: Low-Carb Food Sources   371

FOREWORD

As a physician specializing in sports medicine, I provide a great deal of nutritional counseling to people of all ages, including athletes from the recreational level to the professional level. In my thirteen years of medical training and practice, I've seen a lot of approaches to weight management come and go. Most do not work over the long term, and it is difficult for most dieters to keep any weight loss off, unless they commit to making deep-seated changes in their lifestyle and activity level.

For most of my professional career, I adhered to the generally recognized approach of cutting fat and calories for losing weight. But these types of diets were usually too difficult for most people because of the deprivation that ultimately sabotaged their commitment and discipline. Then along came the low-carbohydrate method of weight management. Though at first skeptical, I nonetheless remained open to any new channel of weight control. I personally tried one of the most popular of these low-carb diets and achieved excellent results. With the exception of athletes (who require higher-carbohydrate diets to fuel themselves for training and competition), I now use some form of low-carbohydrate dieting with most of my patients. I also employ another version of the carbohydrate-controlled diet: low-glycemic diets, which utilize carbohydrates that affect blood sugar and insulin levels less dramatically than other carbohydrates or simple sugars.

The insulin-lowering effect of these diets is essential for allowing the body to burn fat more effectively. Of course, reducing insulin levels appears to help prevent many weight-related diseases, including high cholesterol, hypertension, and diabetes. What's more, recent research suggests that high-carbohydrate diets, particularly when paired with lack of exercise, may now increase the risk of breast cancer.

Carbohydrates make up half of the typical American diet, and in the amounts we consume them (usually in the form of processed carbs and sugar-laden foods), they have become often the leading suspect in our burgeoning national obesity epidemic. Thus, I have come to believe that counting carbohydrates is more important than counting calories. More specifically, counting net carbohydrates is the real key, since the net carbs in food are the ones that have the most measurable impact on blood sugar and insulin levels. Until now, it has been difficult and cumbersome to count net carbs, with no resources to help make this task easy.

Anyone who has been frustrated with having to calculate and count the net carbs in food now has an excellent tool in *The Essential Net Carb Counter*. The information you need to augment your low-carbohydrate diet is contained within this book, with easy access to not only net carbs, but also the calorie and fiber content of foods (both still have an important standing in weight control). I congratulate Dr. Greenwood-Robinson for her latest contribution to the science of nutrition and weight management. It is about time we had a tool like this. So enjoy the book, and get ready to be even more successful in your efforts at low-carbohydrate dieting.

        Robert Monaco, M.D., M.P.H.
        Director of Sports Medicine, Rutgers University
        Clinical Associate Professor, Robert Wood
           Johnson University

INTRODUCTION

Let the Net Carb Countdown Begin!

If you've tried to trim down lately, you're sure to have come across the term *net carbs* on food labels or in diet books. They're a topic of intense interest, especially if your diet of choice is the low-carb variety.

But what exactly are "net carbs"? Do they make a difference? Why is it important to count net carbs? I'll answer these questions and more by decoding the whole net carb issue, so that you can see how they work for you nutritionally.

When a food package lists *net carbs,* it is referring to only the carbohydrates that the body converts to glucose (blood sugar) quickly, such as sugars and starches. Carbohydrates that elevate blood sugar rapidly tend to trigger fat-forming processes in the body, along with other undesirable health effects.

Other carbs, namely dietary fiber and sugar alcohols, do not have the same measurable impact on your blood sugar. Fiber eventually moves out of the body as waste, and sugar alcohols are converted very slowly to blood sugar. So the designation *net carbs* means the total carbohydrate content of food in grams *minus* the grams of fiber and sugar alcohol. For example, if a slice of bread has 7 grams of carbohydrates, with 4 grams of fiber, then the bread contains 3 net grams per slice.

With *The Essential Net Carb Counter*, however, you don't have to do any arithmetic: the net carbs in more than 5,000 foods and food products are already calculated for you. All you have to do is look them up.

Unlike the terms *low-fat* and *low-calorie,* there is not yet any legal definition of what constitutes a "low-carb" food. However, the U.S. Food and Drug Administration (FDA) has announced plans to address this labeling issue and to determine legally what constitutes "low-carb," "reduced-carb," or "carb-free" foods. Some lobbying groups have suggested that a low-carb food should have no more than six grams of carbohydrates per serving and that the term *reduced-carbohydrate* be allowed for foods that have at least 25 percent fewer carbohydrates.

Similarly, the term *net carbs* is not yet a legal classification. But since 2001, the FDA has allowed food manufacturers to use the designation *net carbs* on food labels through a special agreement with the food industry. Other terms for net carbs are *usable carbohydrates, available carbohydrates,* and *nutritive carbohydrates.* So stay tuned; there is more to come on these labeling rules.

Carbohydrates, Net Carbs, Fiber, and Sugar Alcohols

Making up roughly half the calories consumed in the average American diet, carbohydrates are to your body what gas is to a car: the fuel that gets you going. At its most basic, a carbohydrate is a nutrient made up of carbon, hydrogen, and oxygen. Along with fat and protein, it's one of the three "macronutrients" or building blocks of your diet.

During digestion, carbohydrates are broken down into glucose for energy. Assisted by a hormone called insulin, blood glucose is then ushered into cells to be used by various tissues in the body. Carbohydrates therefore nourish your body's tissues, providing energy for your brain, central nervous system, and muscle cells in the form of glucose.

Several things can then happen to glucose in your body. Once inside a cell, it can be quickly metabolized to supply energy. Or it may be converted to either liver or muscle glycogen, the storage form of carbohydrate. When you exercise or use your muscles, your body mobilizes muscle glycogen for energy. Blood glucose can also turn into body fat and get packed away in fat tissue. This happens when you eat more carbohydrates than you need or than your body can store as glycogen. Some blood glucose may also be excreted in your urine.

Carbohydrates are a vital nutrient for good health, supplying the get-up-and-go you need to get up and go, plus providing a bounty of vitamins, minerals, fiber, and other protective nutrients. They are the mainstay of a good diet, provided you keep tabs on how much you take in. Counting net carbs can help you regulate your intake.

Understanding food labels will help you better understand net carbs and how they fit into your overall diet strategy. Depending on the food, food labels list total carbohydrates, sugars, sugar alcohols, and fiber. Each of these types of carbs is metabolized differently in the body.

Total carbohydrates (with the exception of fiber and sugar alcohols) are dismantled into glucose and are absorbed by the body or stored as fat when consumed in large amounts. Sugar—the type found in table sugar, candy, cookies, and baked goods—is very easily and quickly digested in the body. When eaten in excess, sugar has a tendency to be converted into body fat. Sugar is rapidly released into your system, driving your blood sugar up too high and giving you a quick "rush," followed by a fast "crash." The first organ to react to this sugar overload is the pancreas, which responds by secreting more insulin into your bloodstream. Insulin activates fat-cell enzymes, moving fat from the bloodstream into fat cells for storage. Additionally, insulin prevents glucagon (a hormone that opposes the action of insulin) from entering the bloodstream, and glucagon is responsible for unlocking fat stores. The cumulative result of these interactions is the ready conversion of simple sugars to body fat.

Used as artificial sweeteners in many foods, the sugar alcohols include erythritol, hydrogenated starch hydrolysates (HSH), sorbitol, maltitol, lactitol, mannitol, and isomalt. They are derived from fruit or produced from a sugar called dextrose. Most sugar alcohols contain from .2 to 4 calories per gram (sugar provides 4 calories per gram). Sugar alcohols are not digested in the small intestine the way regular sugars are. Instead, they pass straight through to the large intestine where they are broken down by fermentation. As a result, they do not raise blood sugar as much as regular sugar does. For this reason, the sugar alcohols are thought to be better than sugar for people with diabetes. Sugar alcohols also do not promote tooth decay, unlike sugar. However, one downside of sugar alcohols is that, if eaten in excess, they have a laxative effect.

Another sweetener used in many low-carb products is glycerine, a common food additive with a syrupy consistency and sweet taste. Even though glycerine is metabolized in the body like a carbohydrate, it does not turn into blood sugar, or have the same effect on insulin activity that regular carbohydrates do. Glycerine is typically used in packaged foods to prevent them from drying out. This is one reason you find it as an ingredient in so many protein bars.

You probably know all about fiber, an indigestible type of carbohydrate. It's what your grandmother used to call "roughage" and what we know as the stuff in fruits, vegetables, and whole grains that keeps us regular. The "push" response of your intestines depends on adequate fiber in your diet. Low amounts of fiber in the diet are linked to dozens of medical problems, including heart disease, some cancers, diabetes, diverticulosis, and gallstones.

Fiber provides bulk, which is vital for intestinal action. Fiber has an array of health benefits: it improves elimination, flushes cancer-causing substances from the system, and helps normalize cholesterol levels. A diet high in fiber will also help you control your weight in several ways. Fiber makes you feel full, so that you don't overeat. More energy (calories) is spent digesting and absorbing high-fiber foods. In fact, if you increase your fiber intake to 35 grams a day, you'll automatically burn 250 calories a day, without exercising more or eating less. What's more, fiber helps move food through your system more efficiently. This means fewer calories are left to be stored as fat.

Among the fibers used in low-carb food products are a class of additives called fermentable carbohydrates, and they include inulin, resistant starch, and polydextrose. Used in place of higher-carb white flour, these ingredients are fermented in the body the way sugar alcohols are. They provide between 1.6 and 2.5 calories per gram (compared with 4 per gram for regular, higher-carb starches).

The bottom line is that not all carbs are created equal. Some carbs have an impact on your blood sugar, weight, and your overall health, while others do not. Eaten in the right amounts, some carbohydrates—namely, the natural, non-processed types—will help prevent all sorts of life-shortening illnesses, from obesity to heart disease to cancer. Still others (like sugar and junk food) can set into motion harmful biochemical reactions inside your body that incite disease. Restricting the amount of these "bad" carbohydrates in your diet will produce weight loss, lowered blood sugar levels, lowered LDL cholesterol (the artery-clogging type), and reduced triglyceride levels. So if you want to stay healthy and in terrific shape for as long as you can, choose your carbohydrates wisely, and in the right amounts.

Net Carbs and Weight Control

More than two-thirds of the United States population is now considered overweight or obese (weighing 20 percent or more than what is considered a healthy weight), and obesity has become a global epidemic. One of the major nutritional reasons for such widespread (excuse the pun) obesity in America is hiding on the carbohydrate side of the dietary equation. Since low-fat dieting hit the diet scene in the early 1980s, everybody started cutting the fat from their diets while increasing calories from carbohydrates. The diet mantra at the time was "Slash fat, eat carbs." We bought into the low-fat, high-carbohydrate message, but little did we know that we were setting ourselves up for big problems down the road.

Over time, some alarming blips appeared on the nutritional radar screen: people started getting fatter, not thinner. After the government's Food Guide Pyramid (a meal-planning guide now being revised) was introduced in 1991, sermonizing on the value of eating six to eleven servings of carbohydrates a day (including some bad carbs) while eating fats "sparingly," the number of overweight, out-of-shape Americans jumped a whopping 61 percent. We cut the fat from our diets but got wider bottoms and bigger bellies in the process.

Whoa, hold it right there: Aren't you supposed to slash fat to lose weight? Isn't low-fat dieting the ticket to a slender life? Not necessarily, say nutritional scientists who have studied the relationship between the simultaneous rise in obesity and the rise in carbohydrate intake.

INTRODUCTION 7

What appears to be largely responsible for the escalating obesity in our country is that we are eating an excess of bad carbs: foods such as white bread, baked goods, foods with added sugar, and other processed junk foods. The carbohydrate-to-fat ratio in the typical American diet has gotten way out of whack. Bottom line: eating too much of the wrong kinds of carbs—the bad carbs—can make you fat.

So cutting carbs to lose weight makes sense. And low-carb diets do work: when you reduce your intake of carbohydrates, your body starts drawing on its fat reserves for energy. Although your body prefers to fuel itself with carbohydrates, it will use fat as a back-up if necessary.

Metabolically, when you eat bad carbs in excess, your body overproduces insulin in an effort to transport glucose into cells. Medically known as hyperinsulinemia, high concentrations of insulin trigger your body to create more fat cells. Another problem brought on by a diet high in bad carbs is insulin resistance, in which insulin can't do its job of processing sugar and fats for energy. Consequently, your body starts storing more fat than is normal.

Low-carb diets are based on the principle that weight loss is achieved by metabolic and hormonal processes that kick in only when your daily carbohydrate intake falls below a certain level—anywhere from 20 to 80 net carbs a day, depending on the diet. By eating fewer carbs, you keep your blood sugar levels low, and insulin functions as it should: no hyperinsulinemia, no insulin resistance. Your body is able to tap into its fat stores for energy, your weight starts decreasing, and before long you're lean as a hairpin. Studies have begun to show that low-carb dieters lose weight faster than low-fat dieters. So you see, low-carb dieting can be a very efficient way to shed pounds.

Net Carb Cautions

As Americans, we're more carb-conscious than ever—and so are food makers. They've introduced nearly 2,000 reduced-carb foods and beverages into the marketplace in recent years to meet dieters' insatiable demand for low-carb foods. Of these products, more than half fall into four categories: baked goods, confectionary, desserts and ice cream, and snacks.

Red flag warning! With the flood of new processed low-carb products, the attitude to "eat as much as you want as long as it's low-carb" can really pack on pounds, particularly if you're gobbling down a lot of these low-carb packaged foods. Many of these products have nearly as many or more calories as their regular-carb counterparts, despite the net-carb designation on their food labels. For example, a ½-cup serving of regular orange sherbet contains 26 grams of net carbs and 122 calories, whereas half a cup of low-carb orange sherbet provides only 2 net carbs but 174 calories. If you were to fulfill a daily 40-gram net-carb quota (the upper carb limit of many low-carb diets) entirely with low-carb orange sherbet, you'd consume nearly 3,500 calories—enough to make you gain one whole pound!

Just because a carb has minimal impact on your blood sugar doesn't always mean it has minimal impact on your body weight. If you just count carbs, you may lose your weight-loss battle. You must watch your calorie intake, too, because *low-carb* does not mean low-calorie. Overdo these packaged low-carb foods in your diet, and your calories head to the moon—and so do the numbers on your scale.

Also, just because a food is low in net carbs doesn't always mean it's good for you. You still must pay attention to other important nutritional information, such as fiber content. And remember, it's always healthiest in the long run to eat mostly whole foods and populate your diet with fruits, vegetables, and whole-grains, but without going overboard on your total carbohydrate intake.

So although it is important to be a net-carb watcher if you're following a low-carb diet, it is even more important to pay attention to your overall food choices. Here are some suggestions to make sure that your low-carb diet works for you:

- ***Deploy a variety of whole foods rather than processed foods.*** The best—and healthiest—diets contain "good carbs" such as fresh fruits, vegetables, and whole grains. Your body prefers good carbs and uses them so much more efficiently than it uses processed, chemical-laden "bad carbs" such as refined cereals, commercially baked goods, or fat, sugar, and additive-loaded packaged foods. Bad carbs are nutritionally bankrupt and associated with various health problems. Good carbs are bursting with natural fiber, vitamins, minerals, and phytochemicals. You can fill your plate with these foods and still keep your net-carb count in line with what will activate weight loss.

- ***Monitor and increase your fiber intake.*** Fiber is vital for controlling your weight and a top-drawer nutrient for reducing body fat—for several reasons. High-fiber foods make you feel full and thus curb your appetite. In your digestive system, fibers naturally bind to fats you eat and help escort them from the body. The net effect is a reduction in the calories left to be stored as body fat. High-fiber foods require prolonged breakdown and thus release blood sugar more slowly. This action helps prevent dips in blood sugar—dips that can lead to food cravings. A high-fiber diet helps maintain even energy levels throughout the day.

- *Use packaged low-carb foods wisely.* Foods such as low-carb ice cream, candy, snacks, and other items can be higher in calories than some of their regular counterparts (see the discussion below). Use *The Essential Net Carb Counter* to tally calories as well as net carbs, so that you don't eat more calories than required to lose weight.

How to Use *The Essential Net Carb Counter*

The Essential Net Carb Counter is designed as a companion reference source for you if you're following a low-carb diet or a low-calorie diet, or if you just want to monitor carbs, calories, and fiber. It also comes in handy if you eat out a lot, as many Americans do, because it contains the carb and calorie counts of major menu items at some of the most popular restaurant chains in the country.

The food and food products in this counter are alphabetized in food categories as well as under individual categories, so that you'll have no trouble finding whatever you want to look up. If you're looking for a particular food, look for it alphabetically under its category. Let's say you're looking for bagels. Check the table of contents, where you'll find an alphabetized listing of food categories, and go to "Bagels and Bread Products." Turn to the page where these listings begin and go to the *B*'s. Bagels are listed in alphabetical order, so it's easy to locate them. Under "Bagels," you'll find information for low-carb bagels and regular bagels. You can go through the same process to look up any food you want to find. *The Essential Net Carb Counter* contains hundreds of brand-name low-carb foods too. These appear in boldface type for easy access.

The fast-food and restaurant category is arranged for easy use, as well. Foods are categorized alphabetically by food groups such as appetizers, beverages and shakes, breakfast items, desserts, and so forth, and placed under their corresponding restaurant (also listed alphabetically). That way, you can look at each of these foods and compare the carbohydrates and other nutrients of a Burger King selection to a Hardee's selection, for example.

Each food entry lists the following information in this order: food name, serving size, total carbohydrates, net carbs, fiber, and calories, and gives the amount of each in grams or other relevant measurement. Here's a closer look:

Serving Size

One of the reasons Americans are losing the "battle of the bulge" has to do with serving sizes. We've lost track of what a normal serving size looks like. We don't realize that some naturally low-carb foods can dish up far too many calories. If you're to keep your weight in check, you must pay attention to how much you eat. The larger the serving, the more calories the food has in it. This counter defines for you what constitutes a normal, healthy helping. The "serving size" listed refers to the amount of food used by the U.S. Department of Agriculture and the food industry. Stick to these serving sizes, and you're less likely to overindulge.

Total Carbohydrates

The grams of carbohydrates listed in the counter are the total grams of carbohydrates. Although listed separately, the grams of net carbs and fiber are part of the total carbohydrates.

The National Academy of Sciences recommends that adults get 45 percent to 65 percent of their calories from carbohydrates, with a minimum of 130 grams of carbs a day to produce enough glucose for normal brain function. Low-carb diets, of course, recommend far lower intakes of carbohydrates (see below).

Net Carbs

As explained earlier, net carbs refer to the total grams of carbohydrates per serving minus the grams of fiber, sugar alcohol, and other sugar replacers such as glycerine. If you're following a low-carb diet, the net-carb category is one you'll want to zero in on. The optimal number of grams of net carbs per day to trigger weight loss has not been pinpointed conclusively, although most low-carb diets restrict net carbs to between 20 and 80 grams a day.

Fiber

Fiber has a long resume of health benefits, including weight control and protection against many life-shortening diseases. How much fiber should you eat to get its protective benefits? The National Research Council recommends 20 to 35 grams of fiber a day. Your best fiber bets are found in cereals, grains, flours, fruits, certain dinners and entrées, nuts and seeds, vegetables, and some vegetarian-type fast foods. Look for foods that contain at least 2.5 to 3 grams of fiber per serving; such foods are considered "high-fiber."

If you're fiber needy, try to increase your intake gradually. Doing so can help prevent cramping, bloating, and other unpleasant symptoms often associated with increased fiber. Always drink plenty of water, too—eight to ten glasses of pure water daily—because a high-fiber diet is virtually worthless unless there's enough water in your system to help move the food and fiber through.

Calories

These describe the amount of energy provided by one serving and can be used to help you accurately plan your meals if you're following a weight-reducing diet. Generally, most people can lose weight safely by following a diet that supplies 1,200 to 1,500 calories a day. If you use low-carb food products in your diet, be sure to account for the calories they supply.

ABBREVIATIONS AND SYMBOLS

The following table will help you decode the values given for all the entries in *The Essential Net Carb Counter*:

carb	carbohydrate
net carb	net carbohydrate
dia	diameter
fl oz	fluid ounce
g	gram
ml	milliliter
oz	ounce
pkt	packet
serving	serving size identified on food label
t	trace
tbsp	tablespoon
tsp	teaspoon
w/	with
w/o	without
na*	information not available
0 (zero)	no nutrient value

* Note: If *na* appears in a food entry, this does not mean the absence of a particular nutrient, only that analysis of that food for that nutrient is lacking.

All of the nutrient data in *The Essential Net Carb Counter* are based on information from the United States government, from producers of brand-name foods, and from restaurant chains. Scientific journal articles that analyzed the nutrient content of various foods were also consulted.

ALCOHOLIC BEVERAGES

BEER

FOOD	SERVING	TOTAL CARBS (G)	NET CARBS (G)	FIBER (G)	CALORIES
Amber Ice	1 can (12 fl oz)	6	6	0	129
Amstel Light	1 can (12 fl oz)	5	5	0	95
Anheuser Light	1 can (12 fl oz)	7	7	0	91
Arctic Ice	1 can (12 fl oz)	10	10	0	149
Arctic Ice Light	1 can (12 fl oz)	6	6	0	101
Aspen Edge	1 can (12 fl oz)	2.6	2.6	0	94
Beck's	1 can (12 fl oz)	10	10	0	145
Beer, light (generic)	1 can or bottle (12 fl oz)	5	5	0	99
Beer, low carb (generic)	1 can or bottle (12 fl oz)	2.5	2.5	0	96
Beer, regular (generic)	1 can or bottle (12 fl oz)	13	13	0	146
Bud Dry	1 can (12 fl oz)	7.8	7.8	0	130
Bud Light	1 can (12 fl oz)	6.6	6.6	0	110
Bud Ice	1 can (12 fl oz)	8.9	8.9	0	148
Bud Ice Light	1 can (12 fl oz)	6.5	6.5	0	110
Budweiser	1 can (12 fl oz)	10.6	10.6	0	145
Busch	1 can (12 fl oz)	10.2	10.2	0	133
Busch Light	1 can (12 fl oz)	6.7	6.7	0	110
Busch Ice	1 can (12 fl oz)	13	13	0	169
Black Label	1 can (12 fl oz)	8.7	8.7	0	152
Coors	1 can (12 fl oz)	11.3	11.3	0	146
Coors Light	1 can (12 fl oz)	5	5	0	102
Corona Extra	1 can (12 fl oz)	13	13	0	148
Corona Light	1 can (12 fl oz)	6	6	0	105
Heineken	1 can (12 fl oz)	10.8	10.8	0	150

ALCOHOLIC BEVERAGES

FOOD	SERVING	TOTAL CARBS (G)	NET CARBS (G)	FIBER (G)	CALORIES
Keystone Premium	1 can (12 fl oz)	5.6	5.6	0	115
Keystone Light	1 can (12 fl oz)	5	5	0	104
Killian's	1 can (12 fl oz)	13.8	13.8	0	162
Labatt Blue Light	1 can (12 fl oz)	8	8	0	111
Michelob Regular	1 can (12 fl oz)	13.3	13.3	0	155
Michelob Light	1 can (12 fl oz)	7	7	0	113
Michelob ULTRA	1 can (12 fl oz)	2.6	2.6	0	95
Miller Genuine Draft	1 can (12 fl oz)	13.1	13.1	0	154
Miller Light	1 can (12 fl oz)	3.2	3.2	0	96
Natural Light	1 can (12 fl oz)	3.2	3.2	0	95
Old Milwaukee	1 can (12 fl oz)	12.5	12.5	0	145
Old Milwaukee Light	1 can (12 fl oz)	8	8	0	145
Old Milwaukee NA	1 can (12 fl oz)	12	12	0	58
Pabst Blue Ribbon	1 can (12 fl oz)	12	12	0	145
Pabst Blue Ribbon Light	1 can (12 fl oz)	8	8	0	111
Rock Green Light	1 can (12 fl oz)	2.6	2.6	0	92
Samuel Adams Boston Lager	1 can (12 fl oz)	17	17	0	170
Samuel Adams Light	1 can (12 fl oz)	9.7	9.7	0	124
Stroh's	1 can (12 fl oz)	13	13	0	143
Stroh's Light	1 can (12 fl oz)	7	7	0	119
COCKTAIL MIXES					
Cocktail mix, nonalcoholic, concentrated, frozen	1 fl oz	26	26	0	103
Margarita Mix, Desert Lime (Baja Bob's)	4 oz	t	t	0	10
Bloody Mary Mix, Lean & Mean (Baja Bob's)	4 oz	4	4	0	20

ALCOHOLIC BEVERAGES

FOOD	SERVING	TOTAL CARBS (G)	NET CARBS (G)	FIBER (G)	CALORIES
Mai Tai Mix, Maui Madness (Baja Bob's)	4 oz	2	2	0	10
Margarita Mix, Original (Baja Bob's)	4 oz	t	t	0	10
Margarita Mix, Wild Strawberry (Baja Bob's)	4 oz	2	2	0	10
Piña Colada Mix, Crazy Caribe (Baja Bob's)	4 oz	4	0	1	30
Sweet-n-Sour Mix, Loco Lemon (Baja Bob's)	4 oz	1	1	0	10
Whiskey sour mix, powder	1 pkt	17	17	0	65
LIQUEURS					
Amaretto, 56 proof	1 jigger (1.5 fl oz)	25.5	25.5	0	165
Benedictine, 80 proof	1 jigger (1.5 fl oz)	7.5	7.5	0	135
Coffee liqueur, 53 proof	1 jigger (1.5 fl oz)	24	24	0	175
Coffee liqueur, 63 proof	1 jigger (1.5 fl oz)	17	17	0	160
Coffee liqueur w/cream, 34 proof	1 jigger (1.5 fl oz)	10	10	0	154
Cointreau, 80 proof	1 jigger (1.5 fl oz)	10.5	10.5	0	150
Crème de cacao, 54 proof	1 jigger (1.5 fl oz)	22.5	22.5	0	150
Crème de menthe, 72 proof	1 jigger (1.5 fl oz)	21	21	0	181
Drambuie, 80 proof	1 jigger (1.5 fl oz)	13.5	13.5	0	158
Grand Marnier, 80 proof	1 jigger (1.5 fl oz)	10.5	10.5	0	150

ALCOHOLIC BEVERAGES

FOOD	SERVING	TOTAL CARBS (G)	NET CARBS (G)	FIBER (G)	CALORIES
LIQUORS					
Gin, rum, vodka, whiskey, 100 proof	1 jigger (1.5 fl oz)	t	t	0	124
Gin, rum, vodka, whiskey, 80 proof	1 jigger (1.5 fl oz)	t	t	0	97
Gin, rum, vodka, whiskey, 86 proof	1 jigger (1.5 fl oz)	t	t	0	105
Gin, rum, vodka, whiskey, 90 proof	1 jigger (1.5 fl oz)	t	t	0	110
Gin, rum, vodka, whiskey, 94 proof	1 jigger (1.5 fl oz)	t	t	0	116
Hard cider	1 bottle (12 fl oz)	19	19	0	195
MIXED DRINKS					
Bourbon & soda	Standard recipe	1	1	0	110
Daiquiri, canned	1 can (6.8 fl oz)	33	33	0	259
Gin & tonic	Standard recipe	14	14	0	170
Manhattan	Standard recipe	3	3	0	130
Margarita	Standard recipe	4	4	0	170
Martini	Standard recipe	1	1	0	68
Piña colada, canned	1 can (6.8 fl oz)	61	61	t	526
Tequila sunrise, canned	1 can (6.8 fl oz)	24	24	0	232
Tom Collins	Standard recipe	2	2	0	120
Whiskey sour, canned	1 can (6.8 fl oz)	28	28	t	249
WINES					
Wine, dessert, dry	1 glass (3.5 fl oz)	4	4	0	130
Wine, dessert, sweet	1 glass (3.5 fl oz)	12	12	0	158
Wine, table, all varieties	1 glass (3.5 fl oz)	1	1	0	72
Wine, table, red	1 glass (3.5 fl oz)	2	2	0	74
Wine, table, rose	1 glass (3.5 fl oz)	1	1	0	73

FOOD	SERVING	TOTAL CARBS (G)	NET CARBS (G)	FIBER (G)	CALORIES
Wine, table, white	1 glass (3.5 fl oz)	1	1	0	70
WINE COOLERS					
Exotic Berry (Bartles & Jaymes)	1 bottle (12 fl oz)	33	33	0	210
Fuzzy Navel, Tropical Burst (Bartles & Jaymes)	1 bottle (12 fl oz)	38	38	0	230
Margarita, Piña Colada (Bartles & Jaymes)	1 bottle (12 fl oz)	48	48	0	270
Strawberry Daiquiri (Bartles & Jaymes)	1 bottle (12 fl oz)	36	36	0	220

BAGELS AND BREAD PRODUCTS

BAGELS

FOOD	SERVING	TOTAL CARBS (G)	NET CARBS (G)	FIBER (G)	CALORIES
Bagel, cinnamon raisin (Atkins)	1 bagel	20	9	11	200
Bagel, onion (Atkins)	1 bagel	19	8	11	190
Bagel, oat bran, 3"	3" dia	37	34.5	2.5	176
Bagel, plain (Atkins)	1 bagel	18	7	11	190
Bagel, plain, enriched 3"	3" dia	37	35	2	190

BREAD PRODUCTS

FOOD	SERVING	TOTAL CARBS (G)	NET CARBS (G)	FIBER (G)	CALORIES
Bread Crumbs, Original (Keto)	¼ cup	11	4	7	100
Bread Crumbs, Cajun Style (Keto)	¼ cup	11	4	7	100
Bread Crumbs, Italian Style (Keto)	¼ cup	11	4	7	100
Bread Crumbs, Seafood Zest (Keto)	¼ cup	11	4	7	100
Biscuits, buttermilk, refrigerated dough	1 serving	14	14	na	108

BAGELS AND BREAD PRODUCTS

FOOD	SERVING	TOTAL CARBS (G)	NET CARBS (G)	FIBER (G)	CALORIES
Biscuits, buttermilk, refrigerated dough	1 serving, large	25	25	na	195
Biscuit Mix, Buttery Biscuits (MiniCarb)	1 serving (2 oz biscuit)	3	1	2	255
Biscuit Mix, Home Style Country Biscuits (Dixie Diners' Club)	1 biscuit	4	1	3	111
Biscuits, plain, refrigerated dough, higher fat, baked	1 biscuit (2½" dia)	13	13	t	93
Biscuits, plain or buttermilk, prepared from recipe	1 biscuit (4" dia)	45	44	1	358
Biscuits, plain or buttermilk, commercially prepared	1 biscuit, large	37	36	1	280
Cornbread, prepared from dry mix	1 piece	29	28	1	188
Bun Mix (Atkins)	1 bun	4	1	3	23
Bun & Roll Mix, for Hot Dogs/ Hamburger Buns (Dixie Diners' Club)	1 bun	4	1	3	127
Cornbread, prepared from recipe, made w/low-fat (2%) milk	1 piece	28	28	na	173
Dinner rolls (includes brown-and-serve)	1 roll (1 oz)	14	13	1	84
Dinner Roll Mix (Labrada CarbWatchers)	1 serving (17 g)	10	2	5	45
French baguette	1 slice	15	15	t	77

BAGELS AND BREAD PRODUCTS

FOOD	SERVING	TOTAL CARBS (G)	NET CARBS (G)	FIBER (G)	CALORIES
French rolls	1 roll	19	18	1	105
French toast, frozen, ready-to-heat	1 piece	19	18	1	126
Hamburger Rolls, (Wonder)	1 serving	22	21	1	117
Hotdog bun	1 roll	22	21	1	123
Hotdog roll, foot long	1 roll	43	40	3	258
Kaiser rolls	1 roll (3½" dia)	30	29	1	167
Rye dinner roll	1 roll, large (3½"–4" dia)	23	21	2	123
Stuffing, bread	½ cup	22	19	3	178
Stuffing, chicken flavor	½ cup	20	19	1	107
Stuffing, cornbread	½ cup	22	19	3	179
MUFFINS					
Apple Cinnamon, Muffin Mix (MiniCarb)	1 muffin (2 oz)	7	3	4	225
Apple Cinnamon Bran, Muffin Mix (Ketogenics)	1 muffin	10	2	7	190
Banana Nut, Muffin Mix (Atkins)	1 muffin	5	2	3	70
Banana Nut, Muffin Mix (Pure De-lite)	1 muffin (35 g)	6	3	1	110
Blueberry, Muffin & Bread Mix (Flax-O-Meal)	1 muffin	10	3	2	180
Blueberry, Muffin Mix (Pure De-lite)	1 muffin (35 g)	6	3	1	110
Blueberry (New Better)	½ muffin (58 g)	14	5	1	185
Blueberry, commercially prepared	1 large	67	63	4	385

BAGELS AND BREAD PRODUCTS

FOOD	SERVING	TOTAL CARBS (G)	NET CARBS (G)	FIBER (G)	CALORIES
Blueberry, commercially prepared	1 medium	54	51	3	313
Blueberry, commercially prepared	1 small	32	30	2	183
Blueberry, commercially prepared	1 mini	8	8	t	47
Blueberry, prepared from recipe, made w/low-fat milk (2%)	1 muffin	23	23	na	162
Blueberry, toaster type	1 muffin	18	17	1	103
Chocolate (New Better)	½ muffin (58 g)	9	7	1	175
Chocolate Chip, Muffin Mix (Ketogenics)	1 muffin (32 g)	11	1	5	190
Chocolate Chip, Muffin Mix (Atkins)	1 muffin	18	6	2	100
Cinnamon (New Better)	½ muffin (58 g)	14	5.4	1	185
Corn, commercially prepared	1 large	71	66	5	424
Corn, Muffin Mix (Pure De-lite)	1 muffin (35 g)	7	4	1	110
Corn, Deluxe, Muffin Mix (Atkins)	1 muffin	11	8	3	70
Corn, commercially prepared	1 medium	58	54	4	345
Corn, commercially prepared	1 small	34	32	2	201
Corn, commercially prepared	1 mini	9	8	1	52

BAGELS AND BREAD PRODUCTS

FOOD	SERVING	TOTAL CARBS (G)	NET CARBS (G)	FIBER (G)	CALORIES
Corn, prepared from recipe, made w/low-fat milk (2%)	1 muffin (2" dia x 2")	25	25	na	180
Corn, toaster type	1 muffin	19	18	1	114
English muffin, plain, includes sourdough, enriched, w/calcium propionate	1 muffin	26	24	2	134
English muffin, plain, includes sourdough, enriched, w/calcium propionate, toasted	1 muffin	26	25	1	133
English muffin, raisin-cinnamon & apple-cinnamon	1 muffin	28	26	2	139
English muffin, raisin-cinnamon & apple-cinnamon, toasted	1 muffin	28	26	2	137
English muffin, wheat	1 muffin	26	23	3	127
English muffin, whole wheat	1 muffin	27	23	4	134
English muffin, whole wheat, toasted	1 muffin	27	22	5	135
Honey Bran, Muffin Mix (CarbSense)	2 muffins (36 g)	16	5	7	121
Lemon Poppy Seed, Muffin Mix (Pure De-lite)	1 muffin (35 g)	8	3	2	100
Lemon Poppy Seed, Muffin Mix (Atkins)	1 muffin	6	3	3	60

BAGELS AND BREAD PRODUCTS

FOOD	SERVING	TOTAL CARBS (G)	NET CARBS (G)	FIBER (G)	CALORIES
Lemon Poppy Seed, Muffin Mix (New Better)	½ muffin (58 g)	14	5.4	1	185
Mixed grain, includes granola	1 muffin	31	29	2	155
Oat bran	1 small	32	29	3	178
Oat bran	1 mini	8	7	1	46
Oat bran, prepared from recipe, made w/low-fat milk (2%)	1 muffin	24	22	2	169
Orange Cranberry, Muffin Mix (Atkins)	1 muffin	6	2	4	60
Plain, prepared from recipe, made w/low-fat milk (2%)	1 muffin	24	22	2	169
Streusel, Blueberry (New Better)	½ muffin (58 g)	14	5.4	1	185
Streusel, Cinnamon (New Better)	½ muffin (58 g)	14	5.4	1	185
Sweet Corn, Muffin Mix (MiniCarb)	1 muffin (20 oz)	8	2	6	225
Wheat bran, toaster type, w/raisins	1 muffin	19	16	3	106
Wheat bran, toaster type, w/raisins, toasted	1 muffin	19	16	3	106
Wild Strawberry, Muffin Mix (Ketogenics)	1 muffin (32 g)	7	2.5	3.5	215
TORTILLA, WRAPS					
Taco Shells, White Corn (La Tiara)	1 shell (6.6 g)	4	2	2	31

BAGELS AND BREAD PRODUCTS

FOOD	SERVING	TOTAL CARBS (G)	NET CARBS (G)	FIBER (G)	CALORIES
Taco Shells, Yellow Corn (La Tiara)	1 shell (6.6 g)	4	1	3	37
Taco shells, corn, fried	1 medium (5" dia)	13	11	2	98
Tortilla, corn (not fried)	1 medium (6" dia)	9	8	1	42
Tortillas, ready-to-bake or -fry, white flour	1 tortilla (7"–8" dia)	26	25	1	150
Tortillas, ready-to-bake or -fry, white flour	1 tortilla (10" dia)	39	37	2	228
Tortilla, White Flour (Vita's)	1 tortilla, large (73 g)	23	9	14	160
Tortilla, whole wheat	1 medium (7" dia)	23	21	2	84
Tortilla, Whole Wheat (La Superior)	1 tortilla (36 g)	7	4	3	80
Tortilla, Whole Wheat (Mama Lupe's)	1 tortilla (36 g)	7	3	4	60
Tortilla, Whole Wheat (Vita's)	1 tortilla (43 g)	14	5.6	8.4	90
Tortilla, Whole Wheat (La Tortilla Factory)	1 tortilla (36 g)	12	3	9	60
Tortilla, Whole Wheat (La Tortilla Factory)	1 tortilla, large (62 g)	21	6	15	100
Tortilla, Whole Wheat (Vita's)	1 tortilla (43 g)	14	5.6	8.4	90
Tortilla, Whole Wheat (Vita's)	1 tortilla, large (73 g)	23	9	14	160
Tortilla, Whole Wheat, Burrito Size (Adios Carbs)	1 tortilla (47 g)	10	7.5	2.5	108
Tortilla, Whole Wheat, Chocolate Dessert (Adios Carbs)	1 tortilla (38 g)	8	6	2	87

28 BAGELS AND BREAD PRODUCTS

FOOD	SERVING	TOTAL CARBS (G)	NET CARBS (G)	FIBER (G)	CALORIES
Tortilla, Whole Wheat, Green Onion (Adios Carbs)	1 tortilla (38 g)	8	6	2	87
Tortilla, Whole Wheat, Green Onion (La Tortilla Factory)	1 tortilla (36 g)	12	3	9	60
Tortilla, Whole Wheat, Garlic & Herb (Adios Carbs)	1 tortilla (38 g)	8	6	2	87
Tortilla, Whole Wheat, Garlic & Herb (La Tortilla Factory)	1 tortilla (36 g)	12	3	9	60
Tortilla, Whole Wheat, Garlic & Herb (Vita's)	1 tortilla (43 g)	14	5.6	8.4	90
Tortilla, Whole Wheat, Garlic & Herb (Vita's)	1 tortilla, large (73 g)	23	9	14	160
Tortilla, Whole Wheat, Jalapeño Pepper (Adios Carbs)	1 tortilla (38 g)	8	6	2	87
Tortilla, Whole Wheat, Red Chili Pepper (Adios Carbs)	1 tortilla (38 g)	8	6	2	87
Tortilla, Whole Wheat, Regular (Adios Carbs)	1 tortilla (38 g)	8	6	2	87
Tortilla, Whole Wheat, Regular, Restaurant Size (Adios Carbs)	12" tortilla (90 g)	29	21	8	277
Wraps, Brown Rice & Soy Wrap (Atkins)	1 wrap	5	5	0	25
Wraps, Spinach & Soy Wrap (Atkins)	1 wrap	5	5	t	30

BEANS AND LEGUMES

FOOD	SERVING	TOTAL CARBS (G)	NET CARBS (G)	FIBER (G)	CALORIES
Wraps, Tomato, Carrot & Soy Wrap (Atkins)	1 wrap	5	5	t	30
Wraps, Whole Wheat & Soy Wrap (Atkins)	1 wrap	5	5	t	25
BEANS AND LEGUMES					
Adzuki, boiled	½ cup	28	20	8	147
Beans, baked, canned, w/beef	½ cup	22	22	na	161
Beans, baked, canned, w/franks	½ cup	20	11	9	184
Beans, baked, canned, w/pork	½ cup	25	18	7	134
Beans, baked, canned, w/pork & tomato sauce	½ cup	25	19	6	124
Beans, baked, canned, w/pork & sweet sauce	½ cup	27	20	7	140
Beans, baked, canned, plain or vegetarian	½ cup	26	20	6	118
Black beans, boiled	½ cup	20	12.5	7.5	114
Black Beans, Canned, Ranch Style (ConAgra)	½ cup	19	14	5	100
Broadbeans (fava), boiled	½ cup	17	12	5	94
Broadbeans (fava), canned	½ cup	16	11	5	91
Chickpeas (garbanzos), boiled	½ cup	22	16	6	134
Chickpeas (garbanzos), canned	½ cup	27	22	5	143

BEANS AND LEGUMES

FOOD	SERVING	TOTAL CARBS (G)	NET CARBS (G)	FIBER (G)	CALORIES
Cranberry beans, boiled	½ cup	22	13	9	120
Cranberry beans, canned	½ cup	20	14	8	108
Great northern beans, boiled	½ cup	19	13	6	104
Great northern beans, canned	½ cup	28	22	6	149
Kidney beans, boiled	½ cup	20	14	6	112
Kidney beans, canned	½ cup	19	14.5	4.5	104
Lentils, boiled	½ cup	20	22	8	115
Lentils, sprouted, raw	1 cup	17	17	na	82
Lima beans, baby, boiled	½ cup	21	14	7	115
Lima beans, large, boiled	½ cup	20	13	7	108
Lima beans, large, canned	½ cup	18	12	6	95
Mung beans, boiled	½ cup	19	11	8	106
Navy beans, boiled	½ cup	24	18	6	129
Navy beans, canned	½ cup	27	20	7	148
Pink beans, boiled	½ cup	24	19.5	4.5	126
Pinto beans, boiled	½ cup	22	15	7	117
Pinto beans, canned	½ cup	18	12.5	5.5	103
Split peas, boiled	½ cup	21	13	8	116
White beans (small), boiled	½ cup	23	15	9	127
White beans, boiled	½ cup	23	17	6	124
White beans, canned	½ cup	29	23	6	153

FOOD	SERVING	TOTAL CARBS (G)	NET CARBS (G)	FIBER (G)	CALORIES
BEEF					
GROUND					
Ground beef, regular	4 oz	0	0	0	320
Hamburger, 85% lean, pan browned	3 oz	0	0	0	197
Hamburger, 90% lean, pan browned	3 oz	0	0	0	196
Hamburger, 90% lean, broiled	3 oz	0	0	0	173
Hamburger, 95% lean, pan browned	3 oz	0	0	0	164
Hamburger, 95% lean, broiled	3 oz	0	0	0	139
Meat loaf	4 oz	6	5	1	260
CUT					
Bottom round, lean only, trimmed to 0" fat, all grades, roasted	4 oz	0	0	0	207
Bottom round, lean only, trimmed to 0" fat, choice, roasted	4 oz	0	0	0	219
Bottom round, lean only, trimmed to 0" fat, select, roasted	4 oz	0	0	0	194
Bottom round, lean only, trimmed to ¼" fat, all grades, roasted	4 oz	0	0	0	214
Bottom round, lean only, trimmed to ¼" fat, choice, roasted	4 oz	0	0	0	224

BEEF

FOOD	SERVING	TOTAL CARBS (G)	NET CARBS (G)	FIBER (G)	CALORIES
Bottom round, lean only, trimmed to ¼" fat, select, roasted	4 oz	0	0	0	203
Bottom round, lean & fat, trimmed to ⅛" fat, all grades, roasted	4 oz	0	0	0	260
Bottom round, lean & fat, trimmed to ⅛" fat, select, roasted	4 oz	0	0	0	248
Brisket, point half, lean & fat, trimmed to ¼" fat, all grades, braised	4 oz	0	0	0	458
Chuck arm pot roast, lean & fat, trimmed to ½" fat, prime, braised	4 oz	0	0	0	443
Chuck blade roast, lean & fat, trimmed to ½" fat, prime, braised	4 oz	0	0	0	473
Corned beef, canned	4 oz	0	0	0	284
Corned beef loaf, jellied	4 oz	0	0	0	171
Eye of the round, lean only, trimmed to 0" fat, all grades, roasted	4 oz	0	0	0	188
Eye of the round, lean only, trimmed to 0" fat, choice, roasted	4 oz	0	0	0	198
Eye of the round, lean only, trimmed to 0" fat, select, roasted	4 oz	0	0	0	176

FOOD	SERVING	TOTAL CARBS (G)	NET CARBS (G)	FIBER (G)	CALORIES
Eye of the round, lean only, trimmed to ¼" fat, select, roasted	4 oz	0	0	0	181
Eye of the round, lean & fat, trimmed to 0" fat, select, roasted	4 oz	0	0	0	182
Flank steak, lean only, trimmed to 0" fat, choice, broiled	4 oz	0	0	0	235
Flank steak, lean & fat, trimmed to 0" fat, choice, broiled	4 oz	0	0	0	256
Porterhouse steak, lean only, trimmed to 0" fat, all grades, broiled	4 oz	0	0	0	240
Porterhouse steak, lean only, trimmed to 0" fat, choice, broiled	4 oz	0	0	0	254
Porterhouse steak, lean only, trimmed to 0" fat, select, broiled	4 oz	0	0	0	220
Porterhouse steak, lean only, trimmed to ¼" fat, choice, broiled	4 oz	0	0	0	244
Porterhouse steak, lean only, trimmed to ¼" fat, select, broiled	4 oz	0	0	0	230
Retail cuts, fat only, cooked	4 oz	0	0	0	771
Rib, large end (ribs 6–9), lean & fat, trimmed to ⅛" fat, prime, broiled	4 oz	0	0	0	458

BEEF

FOOD	SERVING	TOTAL CARBS (G)	NET CARBS (G)	FIBER (G)	CALORIES
Rib, large end (ribs 6–9), lean & fat, trimmed to ⅛" fat, prime, roasted	4 oz	0	0	0	445
Rib, large end (ribs 6–9), lean & fat, trimmed to ¼" fat, prime, broiled	4 oz	0	0	0	468
Rib, large end (ribs 6–9), lean & fat, trimmed to ¼" fat, prime, roasted	4 oz	0	0	0	456
Rib, large end (ribs 6–9), lean & fat, trimmed to ½" fat, prime, broiled	4 oz	0	0	0	482
Rib, large end (ribs 6–9), lean & fat, trimmed to ½" fat, prime, roasted	4 oz	0	0	0	461
Rib, small end (ribs 10–12), lean & fat, trimmed to ⅛" fat, all grades, broiled	4 oz	0	0	0	374
Rib, small end (ribs 10–12), lean & fat, trimmed to ⅛" fat, all grades, roasted	4 oz	0	0	0	386
Rib, small end (ribs 10–12), lean & fat, trimmed to ⅛" fat, prime, broiled	4 oz	0	0	0	401

FOOD	SERVING	TOTAL CARBS (G)	NET CARBS (G)	FIBER (G)	CALORIES
Rib, small end (ribs 10–12), lean & fat, trimmed to ⅛" fat, prime, roasted	4 oz	0	0	0	466
Rib, small end (ribs 10–12), lean & fat, trimmed to ¼" fat, prime, broiled	4 oz	0	0	0	409
Rib, small end (ribs 10–12), lean & fat, trimmed to ¼" fat, prime, roasted	4 oz	0	0	0	473
Rib, small end (ribs 10–12), lean & fat, trimmed to ½" fat, prime, broiled	4 oz	0	0	0	413
Rib, small end (ribs 10–12), lean & fat, trimmed to ½" fat, prime, roasted	4 oz	0	0	0	476
Rib, whole (ribs 6–12), lean & fat, trimmed to ¼" fat, all grades, broiled	4 oz	0	0	0	388
Rib, whole (ribs 6–12), lean & fat, trimmed to ¼" fat, all grades, roasted	4 oz	0	0	0	406
Rib, whole (ribs 6–12), lean & fat, trimmed to ½" fat, prime, broiled	4 oz	0	0	0	462

BEEF

FOOD	SERVING	TOTAL CARBS (G)	NET CARBS (G)	FIBER (G)	CALORIES
Rib, whole (ribs 6–12), lean & fat, trimmed to ½" fat, prime, roasted	4 oz	0	0	0	482
Round, tip round, lean only, trimmed to 0" fat, all grades, roasted	4 oz	0	0	0	199
Round, tip round, lean only, trimmed to 0" fat, choice, roasted	4 oz	0	0	0	204
Round, tip round, lean only, trimmed to 0" fat, select, roasted	4 oz	0	0	0	193
Round, tip round, lean only, trimmed to ¼" fat, all grades, roasted	4 oz	0	0	0	210
Round, tip round, lean only, trimmed to ¼" fat, choice, roasted	4 oz	0	0	0	213
Round, tip round, lean only, trimmed to ¼" fat, select, roasted	4 oz	0	0	0	204
Round, tip round, lean & fat, trimmed to 0" fat, all grades, roasted	4 oz	0	0	0	216
Round, tip round, lean & fat, trimmed to 0" fat, choice, roasted	4 oz	0	0	0	227

FOOD	SERVING	TOTAL CARBS (G)	NET CARBS (G)	FIBER (G)	CALORIES
Round, tip round, lean & fat, trimmed to 0" fat, select, roasted	4 oz	0	0	0	211
Round, tip round, lean & fat, trimmed to 1/8" fat, all grades, roasted	4 oz	0	0	0	248
Round, tip round, lean & fat, trimmed to 1/8" fat, all grades, roasted	4 oz	0	0	0	258
Round, tip round, lean & fat, trimmed to 1/8" fat, all grades, roasted	4 oz	0	0	0	238
Sandwich steaks	4 oz	0	0	0	346
Short ribs, lean & fat, choice, braised	4 oz	0	0	0	534
T-bone steak, lean only, trimmed to 0" fat, all grades, broiled	4 oz	0	0	0	214
T-bone steak, lean only, trimmed to 0" fat, choice, broiled	4 oz	0	0	0	224
T-bone steak, lean only, trimmed to 0" fat, select, broiled	4 oz	0	0	0	201
T-bone steak, lean only, trimmed to 1/4" fat, all grades, broiled	4 oz	0	0	0	229

BEEF

FOOD	SERVING	TOTAL CARBS (G)	NET CARBS (G)	FIBER (G)	CALORIES
T-bone steak, lean only, trimmed to ¼" fat, choice, broiled	4 oz	0	0	0	232
T-bone steak, lean only, trimmed to ¼" fat, select, broiled	4 oz	0	0	0	224
Tenderloin, lean only, trimmed to 0" fat, choice, broiled (filet mignon, beef medallions)	4 oz	0	0	0	240
Top round, lean only, trimmed to 0" fat, all grades, braised (London broil)	4 oz	0	0	0	226
Top round, lean & fat, trimmed to 0" fat, choice, braised (London broil)	4 oz	0	0	0	245
Top round, lean only, trimmed to 0" fat, select, braised (London broil)	4 oz	0	0	0	215
Top round, lean & fat, trimmed to 0" fat, select, braised (London broil)	4 oz	0	0	0	227
Top round, lean only, trimmed to ¼" fat, all grades, braised (London broil)	4 oz	0	0	0	231

FOOD	SERVING	TOTAL CARBS (G)	NET CARBS (G)	FIBER (G)	CALORIES
Top round, lean only, trimmed to ¼" fat, all grades, broiled (London broil)	4 oz	0	0	0	204
Top round, lean & fat, trimmed to ⅛" fat, select, broiled (London broil)	4 oz	0	0	0	222
Top sirloin, lean only, trimmed to 0" fat, all grades, broiled	4 oz	0	0	0	216
Top sirloin, lean only, trimmed to 0" fat, choice, broiled	4 oz	0	0	0	227
Top sirloin, lean only, trimmed to 0" fat, select, broiled	4 oz	0	0	0	204
Top sirloin, lean only, trimmed to ¼" fat, all grades, broiled	4 oz	0	0	0	221
Top sirloin, lean only, trimmed to ¼" fat, choice, broiled	4 oz	0	0	0	229
Top sirloin, lean only, trimmed to ¼" fat, select, broiled	4 oz	0	0	0	211
Top sirloin, lean & fat, trimmed to 0" fat, all grades, broiled	4 oz	0	0	0	244
Top sirloin, lean & fat, trimmed to 0" fat, choice, broiled	4 oz	0	0	0	260

40 BREAD

FOOD	SERVING	TOTAL CARBS (G)	NET CARBS (G)	FIBER (G)	CALORIES
Top sirloin, lean & fat, trimmed to 0" fat, select, broiled	4 oz	0	0	0	221
VARIETY MEATS, LEAN					
Beef heart, simmered	4 oz	0	0	0	200
Beef kidneys, simmered	4 oz	1	1	0	163
Beef liver, braised	4 oz	4	4	0	182
BREAD					
BREAD					
Cinnamon Raisin Bread (CarbXtract)	1 slice	6	4.5	1.5	42
Cinnamon Raisin Swirl Bread (CarbXtract)	1 slice	6	4.5	1.5	51
Cornmeal Crusted Round Bread (CarbXtract)	1 slice	6	4.5	1.5	42
Cracked wheat bread	1 slice	12	10.6	1.4	65
Egg bread	1 slice	19	18	1	115
French Bread (CarbXtract)	1 slice	6	4.5	1.5	42
French Round Bread (CarbXtract)	1 slice	6	4.5	1.5	42
Italian bread	1 slice, large (4½" x 3¼" x ¾")	15	14	1	81
Italian Bread, Garlic, Crusty (Pepperidge Farm)	1 serving	21	21	na	186
Mixed-grain bread	1 slice	12	10	2	65
Multigrain Bread (Atkins)	1 slice	7	3	4	70

FOOD	SERVING	TOTAL CARBS (G)	NET CARBS (G)	FIBER (G)	CALORIES
Multigrain Bread (CarbXtract)	1 slice	6	4.5	1.5	42
Oat bran bread	1 slice	12	11	1	71
Oat bran bread, reduced calorie	1 slice	10	7	3	46
Oatmeal bread	1 slice	13	12	1	73
Oatmeal bread, reduced calorie	1 slice	10	10	na	48
Pita bread, whole wheat	4" dia	15	13	2	74
Protein bread	1 slice	8	7	1	47
Pumpernickel bread	1 slice	12	10	2	65
Pumpernickel Bread (CarbXtract)	1 slice	6	4.5	1.5	42
Raisin bread	1 slice	14	13	1	71
Rice bran bread	1 slice	12	11	1	66
Rye bread	1 slice	15	13	2	83
Rye bread, reduced calorie	1 slice	9	6	3	47
Rye Bread (Atkins)	1 slice	7	3	4	70
Rye Round Bread (CarbXtract)	1 slice	6	4.5	1.5	42
Sourdough Bread (CarbXtract)	1 slice	6	4.5	1.5	42
Sourdough Round Bread (CarbXtract)	1 slice	6	4.5	1.5	42
Wheatberry bread	1 slice	12	11	1	65
Wheat bran bread	1 slice	17	15.6	1.4	89
Wheat bread, reduced calorie	1 slice	10	7	3	46

42 BREAD

FOOD	SERVING	TOTAL CARBS (G)	NET CARBS (G)	FIBER (G)	CALORIES
Wheat Bread (CarbXtract)	1 slice	6	4.5	1.5	42
Wheat/Pumpernickel (Marble) Bread (CarbXtract)	1 slice	6	4.5	1.5	42
Wheat germ bread	1 slice	13.5	12.5	t	73
White Bread, Country White (Atkins)	1 slice	7	3	4	70
White bread	1 slice	12	12	t	67
Whole wheat bread	1 slice	13	11	2	69
"X" Bread (CarbXtract)	1 slice	7	5	2	69
"X" Cinnamon Raisin Bread (CarbXtract)	1 slice	7	5	2	76
BREAD MIXES					
Banana Bread Mix (Keto)	⅜" slice	3	2	1	70
Caraway Rye Bread Mix (Atkins)	½" slice	8	3	5	70
Cinnamon Raisin Bread Mix (Keto)	½" slice	5	3	2	70
Country White Bread Mix (MiniCarb)	1 slice (18 g)	7	3	4	80
Country White Bread Mix (Atkins)	½" slice	8	3	5	70
French Loaf Bread Mix (Keto)	½" slice	5	2	3	70
Golden Original Bread Mix (Keto)	⅜" slice	3	2	1	70
Harvest Wheat Bread Mix (CarbSense)	1 slice (18 g)	4	3	1	60

FOOD	SERVING	TOTAL CARBS (G)	NET CARBS (G)	FIBER (G)	CALORIES
Honey Wheat Bread Mix (Ketogenics)	1 slice	7	2	5	80
Pumpernickel Bread Mix (Keto)	⅜" slice	3	2	1	70
Pumpernickel Rye Bread Mix (Ketogenics)	1 slice	7	2	5	80
Rye Bread Mix (Keto)	⅜" slice	3	2	1	70
Sourdough Bread Mix (Atkins)	½" slice	8	3	5	70
Sourdough Rye Bread Mix (Keto)	½" slice	5	2	3	70
Wheat Bread Mix (CarboRite)	¼" slice	4	4	0	55
Wheat Bread Mix (Labrada CarbWatchers)	1 slice (0.5 oz)	7	4	3	40
Wheat Bread Mix (Ketogenics)	1 slice	6	2	4	80
Whole Wheat Bread Mix (Nature's Own)	1 slice (1 oz)	7	5	2	60

CAKE

CAKES BY BRAND

FOOD	SERVING	TOTAL CARBS (G)	NET CARBS (G)	FIBER (G)	CALORIES
Atkins Almond Crème Coffee Cake Mix	1 piece (1/12 of 20 oz cake)	5	4	1	46
Atkins Cheesecake Mix	1 slice (3.5 oz)	2	1	1	11
Atkins Cheesecake, Pumpkin (Frozen)	1 slice (3 oz)	3	3	0	210
Atkins Chocolate & Buttercream, Celebration Cake	1 slice (2.25 oz)	17	1	2	254

44 CAKE

FOOD	SERVING	TOTAL CARBS (G)	NET CARBS (G)	FIBER (G)	CALORIES
Atkins Chocolate Cake Roll w/Chocolate Filling	1 slice (2.6 oz)	6	5	1	230
Atkins Chocolate Cake Roll w/Strawberry Filling	1 slice (2.6 oz)	5	4	1	220
Atkins Devil's Food Cake Mix	1 piece (2 oz)	5	4	1	35
Atkins Chocolate Truffle Tort	2.25 oz	18	2	3	274
Atkins Lemon Chiffon Tort	2 oz	15	2	2	169
Dixie Diners' Club Almond Crème Coffee Cake Mix	1 piece (1/12 of cake)	5	4	1	186
Dixie Diners' Club Cheesecake Mix	1 slice (3.5 oz)	2	1	1	214
Dixie Diners' Club Devil's Food Cake Mix	1 piece (1/12 of cake)	5	4	1	225
Gare's Cheesecake Mix, New York Style	1 slice (23 g)	25	1	1	120
Hostess Ding Dongs Chocolate Snack Cake, Crème Filling	1 serving	45	43	2	368
Labrada CarbWatchers Chocolate Cake & Muffin Mix	1 serving (12 g)	9	3	2	80
Labrada CarbWatchers Yellow Crème Cake & Muffin Mix	1 serving (12 g)	9	3	2	80

FOOD	SERVING	TOTAL CARBS (G)	NET CARBS (G)	FIBER (G)	CALORIES
MiniCarb Carrot Cake Mix	1 slice (⅑ of cake)	10	4	6	280
MiniCarb Chocolate Cake Mix	1 slice (⅑ of cake)	16	4	12	230
Nabisco Snackwell's Devil's Food Cookie Cakes, Fat Free	1 serving	12	12	t	49
Wise CHOice Cheesecake Mix Made w/Cream Cheese	1 slice (⅛ of cake)	4	0	4	220
Wise CHOice Cheesecake Mix Made w/Neufchâtel Cheese	1 slice (⅛ of cake)	4	0	4	170
Wise CHOice Cheesecake Mix Made w/Philadelphia Fat-Free Cream Cheese	1 slice (⅛ of cake)	4	0	4	85
CAKES, GENERIC					
Angel food cake, commercially prepared	1 piece (1/12 of 12 oz cake)	16	16	t	72
Boston cream pie, commercially prepared	1 piece (⅙ of pie)	39	39	1	232
Cherry fudge cake w/chocolate frosting	1 piece (⅛ of cake)	27	26	1	187
Chocolate cake, commercially prepared	1 piece (⅛ of 18 oz cake)	35	33	2	235
Fruitcake, commercially prepared	1 piece	26	24	2	139

46 CAKE

FOOD	SERVING	TOTAL CARBS (G)	NET CARBS (G)	FIBER (G)	CALORIES
Gingerbread cake, prepared from recipe	1 piece (1/9 of 8" square)	36	36	na	263
Pineapple upside-down cake, prepared from recipe	1 piece (1/9 of 8" square)	58	57	1	367
Pound cake, commercially prepared, butter	1 piece (1/12 of 12 oz cake)	14	14	t	109
Pound cake, commercially prepared, other than all butter, unenriched	1 piece (1/12 of 12 oz cake)	15	15	t	109
Shortcake, biscuit type, prepared from recipe	2 oz	28	28	na	196
Snack cakes, crème-filled, chocolate w/frosting	1 cupcake	30	30	t	188
Snack cakes, crème-filled, sponge	1 cupcake	27	27	t	157
Snack cakes, cupcakes, chocolate, w/frosting, low fat	1 cupcake	29	27	2	131
Sponge cake, commercially prepared	1 piece (1/12 of 16 oz cake)	23	23	t	110
Sponge cake, prepared from recipe	1 piece (1/12 of 16 oz cake)	36	36	na	187
White cake, prepared from recipe, w/coconut frosting	1 piece (1/12 of 9" dia cake)	71	70	1	399

FOOD	SERVING	TOTAL CARBS (G)	NET CARBS (G)	FIBER (G)	CALORIES
White cake, prepared from recipe, w/o frosting	1 piece (1/12 of 9" dia cake)	42	41	1	264
Yellow cake, commercially prepared, w/chocolate frosting	1 piece (1/8 of 18 oz cake)	35	35	1	243
Yellow cake, commercially prepared, w/vanilla frosting	1 piece (1/8 of 18 oz cake)	38	38	t	239
Yellow cake, prepared from recipe, w/o frosting	1 piece (1/8 of 8" dia cake)	36	36	t	245

CANDY

CANDY, GENERIC, ALL TYPES

FOOD	SERVING	TOTAL CARBS (G)	NET CARBS (G)	FIBER (G)	CALORIES
Almond & coconut candy bar	1 package (1.76 oz)	29	26	3	235
Almond & coconut candy bar	1 bar snack size	11	10	1	91
Butterscotch candy	3 pieces	14	14	0	63
Caramel candy bar	1 bar (1.25 oz)	22	22	t	162
Caramel candy bar	1 bar (1.6 oz)	29	28	1	208
Caramel candy	1 piece	8	8	t	39
Caramel cookie bars	1 package (2 oz)	37	36	1	284
Caramel cookie bars	2 bars (2.06 oz)	38	37	1	289
Caramels in milk chocolate	1 pkt (1.91 oz)	37	37	t	256
Caramels in milk chocolate	2 rolls (3 pieces per roll)	25	25	t	171

CANDY

FOOD	SERVING	TOTAL CARBS (G)	NET CARBS (G)	FIBER (G)	CALORIES
Caramels in milk chocolate	7 pieces	28	28	t	199
Carob candy bar	1 bar (3 oz)	49	46	3	470
Chocolate-covered coconut candy bar	1 bar, snack size	11	10	1	92
Chocolate-covered coconut candy bar	1 pkt (1.9 oz)	31	29	2	258
Chocolate fudge, prepared from recipe	1 piece	13	13	t	70
Chocolate nougat bar	1 bar (0.8 oz)	18	18	t	96
Chocolate nougat bar	1 bar (1.813 oz)	39	38	1	212
Chocolate nougat bar	1 bar, fun size	13	13	t	71
Chocolate wafer bar	1 bar, miniature (0.35 oz)	6	6	t	52
Chocolate wafer bar	1 bar (1.5 oz)	27	26	1	217
Chocolate wafer bar	1 bar (1.625 oz)	30	29	1	238
Chocolate wafer bar	1 bar (2.8 oz)	50	48	2	403
Chocolate wafer bar	1 bar (3.375 oz)	62	60	2	496
Dark chocolate bar	1 bar (1.45 oz)	24	21	3	218
Dark chocolate bar	1 bar (2.6 oz)	43	38	5	388
Dinner mints	1 piece	6	6	t	29
Dinner mints	5 pieces	31	30	1	147
Fruit chews	1 pkt, fun size	35	35	0	166
Fruit chews	1 pkt (2.07 oz)	49	49	0	234
Fruit chews	1 serving	34	34	0	158
Gumdrops	10 gumdrops	36	36	0	139
Gumdrops	1 cup of gumdrops	180	180	0	703
Gummy bears	10 gummy bears	22	22	0	85
Jelly beans	10 small	10	10	0	40

CANDY

FOOD	SERVING	TOTAL CARBS (G)	NET CARBS (G)	FIBER (G)	CALORIES
Jelly beans	10 large (1 oz)	26	26	0	103
Marshmallows, miniature	10 pieces	6	6	0	22
Marshmallows, miniature	1 cup	41	41	0	159
Marshmallows, regular	1 piece	6	6	0	23
Milk chocolate–coated peanuts	10 pieces	20	18	2	208
Milk chocolate–coated peanuts	1 cup	74	67	7	773
Milk chocolate–coated raisins	10 pieces	7	6	t	39
Milk chocolate–coated raisins	1 cup	123	115	8	702
Milk chocolate bar, miniature	1 bar	4	4	t	36
Milk chocolate bar	1 bar (1.55 oz)	26	24	2	226
Milk chocolate bar w/almonds	1 bar (1.45 oz)	22	19	3	216
Milk chocolate bar w/almonds	1 bar (1.55 oz)	23	20	3	231
Milk chocolate bar w/rice cereal	1 bar, miniature	6	6	t	50
Milk chocolate bar w/rice cereal	1 bar (1.4 oz)	25	24	1	198
Milk chocolate bar w/rice cereal	1 bar (1.45 oz)	29	28	1	223
Milk chocolate bar w/rice cereal	1 bar (1.55 oz)	28	27	1	218
Milk chocolate bar w/rice cereal	1 bar (1.65 oz)	30	28	2	233

CANDY

FOOD	SERVING	TOTAL CARBS (G)	NET CARBS (G)	FIBER (G)	CALORIES
Peanut bar	1 bar (1.4 oz)	19	17	2	209
Peanut bar	1 bar (1.6 oz)	21	18	3	235
Peanut butter candies pieces	¼ cup	28	27	1	234
Peanut butter candies pieces	10 pieces	5	4	t	40
Peanut butter candies pieces	1 pkt (1.63 oz)	28	27	1	229
Peanut butter cookie bars	2 bars (1.89 oz)	28	26	2	286
Peanut butter cups	1 piece miniature	4	4	t	36
Peanut butter cups	1 cup (0.6 oz)	9	8	1	88
Peanut butter cups	2 cups (1.6 oz)	25	23	2	232
Peanut chocolate candies	1 cup	103	97	6	877
Peanut chocolate candies	1 pkt, fun size	13	12	1	108
Peanut chocolate candies	1 pkt (1.67 oz)	28	26	2	243
Peanut chocolate candies	1 pkt (1.74 oz)	30	28	2	253
Peppermint patty	1 patty (1.5 oz)	35	34	1	165
Plain chocolate candies	1 cup	148	143	5	1023
Plain chocolate candies	1 box (1.48 oz)	30	29	1	207
Plain chocolate candies	1 pkt (1.69 oz)	34	33	1	236
Peppermints mints	3 pieces	15	15	na	59
Semisweet chocolate	1 cup chips (6 oz pkt)	106	96	10	805
Semisweet chocolate	1 cup of mini chips	109	99	10	829
Semisweet chocolate	1 oz or 60 pieces	18	16	2	136

CANDY

FOOD	SERVING	TOTAL CARBS (G)	NET CARBS (G)	FIBER (G)	CALORIES
Toffee bar	1 bar (1.4 oz)	24	24	t	209
Sugar-coated almonds	6 pieces	15	14	1	96
Sweet chocolate bar	1 bar (1.45 oz)	24	22	2	207
Strawberry twists candy	4 pieces from 5 oz pkt	30	30	0	556
Strawberry twists candy	4 pieces from 8 oz pkt	36	36	0	659

CANDY, BY BRAND NAME, CHOCOLATE & CHOCOLATE BARS, LOW CARB

FOOD	SERVING	TOTAL CARBS (G)	NET CARBS (G)	FIBER (G)	CALORIES
Asher's Almond Buttercrunch	2 pieces (40 g)	22	1	2	120
Asher's Cherry Cordials	2 pieces (40 g)	28	5	0	140
Asher's Chocolate Bunny	1 bunny	24	1	1	190
Asher's Chocolate Duck	1 duck	21	2	t	170
Asher's Dark Chocolate Flavored Bar	1 bar (47 g)	25	2	3	230
Asher's Chocolate Nut Fudge Egg	⅓ egg (40 g)	23.4	2	1	170
Asher's Coconut Cream Egg	⅓ egg (40 g)	24.6	1.7	t	180
Asher's Liquid Caramel Bar	1 bar (47 g)	29	2	t	200
Asher's Liquid Raspberry Bar	1 bar (47 g)	31	1	4	190
Asher's Milk Chocolate Flavored Bar	1 bar (47 g)	27	6	2	220
Asher's Pecan & Caramel Bar	1 bar (47 g)	29	2	t	210

52 CANDY

FOOD	SERVING	TOTAL CARBS (G)	NET CARBS (G)	FIBER (G)	CALORIES
Asher's Pecan Caramel Patties	2 pieces (40 g)	20	1	1	210
Asher's Peanut Butter Cups	3 cups (41 g)	21	2	1	200
Asher's Peanut Butter Meltaway Egg	⅓ egg (40 g)	17	2	2	210
Asher's Peanut Butter Truffle Bar	1 bar (47 g)	23	2	2	230
Asher's Peanut Clusters	4 pieces (41 g)	20	2	1	200
Asher's Peppermint Patties	2 pieces (41 g)	28	0	3	150
Asher's Truffle Bar	1 bar (47 g)	31	2	t	200
Asher's Vanilla Butter Cream Egg	⅓ egg (40 g)	27	1.1	0	140
Asher's Vanilla Caramels	2 pieces (40 g)	27	0	5	130
Atkins Endulge Chocolate Candy Bar	1 bar (30 g)	2	2	3	150
Atkins Endulge Chocolate Crunch Candy Bar	1 bar (30 g)	2	2	3	150
Atkins Endulge Caramel Nut Chew	1 bar (1.23 oz)	17	2	t	140
Atkins Endulge Peanut Butter Cups	3 cups	17	2	0	160
CarboRite Candy Coated Chocolate	1 bag	24	1	5	120
CarboRite Caramel Bar	1 bar (28.5 g)	18	0	0	100
CarboRite Caramel Nougat Bar	1 bar (28.5 g)	20	0	1	100

CANDY

FOOD	SERVING	TOTAL CARBS (G)	NET CARBS (G)	FIBER (G)	CALORIES
CarboRite Crispy Caramel Bar	1 bar (28.5 g)	15	0	0	130
CarboRite Chocolate Almond Bar	1 bar (28 g)	13	1	6	120
CarboRite Chocolate Almond Bar	1 bar (50 g)	25	2	1	230
CarboRite Chocolate Coconut Bar	1 bar (32 g)	17	0	2	110
CarboRite Chocolate Coconut & Almonds Bar	1 bar (32 g)	17	1	2	120
CarboRite Chocolate-Covered Peanuts	1 bag	18	3	5	150
CarboRite Chocolate Crisp Bar	1 bar (28 g)	14	2	6	110
CarboRite Chocolate Crisp Bar	2 pieces (7 g)	.4	0	t	36
CarboRite Chocolate Mint Bar	1 bar (28 g)	15	1	7	110
CarboRite Chocolate Peanut Butter Bar	1 bar (28 g)	14	1	5	120
CarboRite Chocolate Peanut Butter Bar	1 bar (50 g)	27	1	2	250
CarboRite Dark Chocolate Bar, Small Size	2 pieces (7 g)	.4	0	.4	37
CarboRite Chocolate Truffle Bar	1 bar (28 g)	15	1	5	100
CarboRite Chocolate Truffle Bar	1 bar (50 g)	30	2	2	190

54 CANDY

FOOD	SERVING	TOTAL CARBS (G)	NET CARBS (G)	FIBER (G)	CALORIES
CarboRite Peanut Butter Cup	1 cup (35 g)	17	t	t	170
CarboRite Peanut Caramel Bar	1 bar (28.5 g)	20	0	1	110
CarboRite Pecan Cluster Bar	1 bar (28.5 g)	15	t	t	120
CarboRite Toffee Bar	1 bar (28.5 g)	15	0	0	110
Carb Slim Bites, Peanut Butter	1 serving (29 g)	14	0	6	114
Carb Slim Bites, Chocolate Caramel	1 serving (29 g)	14	0	6	118
Doctor's CarbRite Diet Sugar Free Bar, Cookies 'n Cream	1 piece (7 g)	4	0	0	32
Doctor's CarbRite Diet Sugar Free Bar, Dark Chocolate	1 piece (7 g)	4	0	.5	31
Doctor's CarbRite Diet Sugar Free Bar, Dark Chocolate w/Almonds	1 piece (7 g)	4	0	1	33
Doctor's CarbRite Diet Sugar Free Bar, Milk Chocolate	1 piece (7 g)	4	0	0	32
Doctor's CarbRite Diet Sugar Free Bar, Milk Chocolate w/Peanuts	1 piece (7 g)	3	0	0	33
Doctor's CarbRite Diet Sugar Free Bar, Milk Chocolate w/Soy Crisps	1 piece (7 g)	3	0	.5	30

CANDY

FOOD	SERVING	TOTAL CARBS (G)	NET CARBS (G)	FIBER (G)	CALORIES
Doctor's CarbRite Diet Sugar Free Bar, Mint Chocolate	1 piece (7 g)	4	0	.5	31
Doctor's CarbRite Diet Sugar Free Bar, White Chocolate	½ piece (7 g)	0	0	0	32
Ketogenics Chocolate Almond Bar	1 bar (50 g)	25	2	2	250
Ketogenics Chocolate Crisp Bar	1 bar (50 g)	26	2	1	240
Labrada CarbWatchers Chocolate Bar, Hazelnut Crisp	1 serving (14 g)	8	0	0	80
Labrada CarbWatchers Chocolate Bar, Oranges & Crème	1 serving (14 g)	8	0	0	80
Labrada CarbWatchers Chocolate Bar, Pistachio Crème	1 serving (14 g)	8	0	0	80
Labrada CarbWatchers Chocolate Bar, Praline Mocha	1 serving (14 g)	7	0	0	80
Labrada CarbWatchers Chocolate Bar, Raspberry & Crème	1 serving (14 g)	8	1.5	0	80
Labrada CarbWatchers Chocolate Bar, Vanilla Crème	1 serving (14 g)	8	0	0	80
La Nouba Dark Chocolate Bar	1 bar (1.5 oz)	19.2	1.1	4.2	190
La Nouba Milk Chocolate Bar	1 bar (1.5 oz)	21	3.7	1.1	204

56 CANDY

FOOD	SERVING	TOTAL CARBS (G)	NET CARBS (G)	FIBER (G)	CALORIES
La Nouba Milk Chocolate Almond Bar	1 bar (1.5 oz)	19.6	3.5	4.2	210
La Nouba Milk Chocolate Coconut Bar	1 bar (1.5 oz)	21	3.7	1.1	204
La Nouba Milk Chocolate Mint Bar	1 bar (1.5 oz)	21	3.7	1.1	204
La Nouba Milk Chocolate Raspberry Bar	1 bar (1.5 oz)	21	3.7	1	204
La Nouba Silhouette, Coconut Cream	1 bar (0.64 oz)	8.8	1.4	t	72
La Nouba Silhouette, Lemon Cream	1 bar (0.64 oz)	8.8	1.4	t	72
La Nouba Silhouette, Orange Cream	1 bar (0.64 oz)	8.8	1.4	t	72
La Nouba Silhouette, Vanilla Cream	1 bar (0.64 oz)	8.8	1.4	t	72
La Nouba White Chocolate Bar	1 bar (1.5 oz)	22.9	3.5	1.1	205
Lean Protein Bites, Milk Chocolate Covered Crunch	1 bag	1	1	0	120
Lean Protein Bites, White Chocolate Covered Crunch	1 bag	1	1	0	120
Low Carb Success Sugar Free Milk Chocolate Baking Chips	1 serving (1 oz)	18	1	1	130

CANDY

FOOD	SERVING	TOTAL CARBS (G)	NET CARBS (G)	FIBER (G)	CALORIES
Low Carb Success Sugar Free Semi-sweet Chocolate Baking Chips	1 serving (1 oz)	18	1	2	131
Low Carb Success Sugar Free Chocolate Baking Chips	1 oz	18	1	1	130
Pure De-lite Almond Bar	1 bar (28 g)	14	1	2	110
Pure De-lite Caramel Bar	1 bar (28 g)	19	2	1	120
Pure De-lite Caramel Crisp Bar	1 bar (28 g)	18	2	1	120
Pure De-lite Caramel Nougat Bar	1 bar (28 g)	20	1	1	110
Pure De-lite Caramel Peanut Butter Bar w/Peanuts	1 bar (28 g)	17	2	1	120
Pure De-lite Caramel Pecan Bar	1 bar (28 g)	17	2	1	130
Pure De-lite Coconut Bar	1 bar (28 g)	13	0	2	110
Pure De-lite Dark Chocolate Bar	1 bar (38 g)	22	0	2	170
Pure De-lite Dark Milk Chocolate, Treasure Bite	1 bar (12 g)	.4	0	1.2	55
Pure De-lite Dark Chocolate Mint, Chewy Sensation	1 bar (32 g)	4	3	1	106

58 CANDY

FOOD	SERVING	TOTAL CARBS (G)	NET CARBS (G)	FIBER (G)	CALORIES
Pure De-lite Milk Chocolate, Treasure Bite	1 bar (12 g)	1.1	.7	t	59
Pure De-lite Milk Chocolate Almond, Treasure Bite	1 bar (12 g)	1.3	.8	t	61
Pure De-lite Milk Chocolate Crisp, Treasure Bite	1 bar (12 g)	1.6	1.3	t	56
Pure De-lite Milk Chocolate Caramel, Chewy Sensation	1 bar (32 g)	4.6	4.2	t	109
Pure De-lite Milk Chocolate Mocha, Chewy Sensation	1 bar (32 g)	4.6	4.2	t	109
Pure De-lite Milk Chocolate Bar	1 bar (38 g)	21	3	1	190
Pure De-lite Milk Chocolate w/ Almonds Bar	1 bar (38 g)	22	3	2	190
Pure De-lite Milk Chocolate w/ Coconut Bar	1 bar (38 g)	na	2.6	na	190
Pure De-lite Milk Chocolate w/ Crisps Bar	1 bar (38 g)	21	3	1	190
Pure De-lite Milk Chocolate w/ Mint Bar	1 bar (38 g)	3.4	2.3	1.1	187
Pure De-lite Milk Chocolate w/ Orange Bar	1 bar (38 g)	3.4	2.3	1.1	187

CANDY

FOOD	SERVING	TOTAL CARBS (G)	NET CARBS (G)	FIBER (G)	CALORIES
Pure De-lite Milk Chocolate w/ Peanuts Bar	1 bar (38 g)	3.7	2.6	1	190
Pure De-lite Mint Patty	1 patty (28 g)	20	0	1	80
Pure De-lite Peanut Butter Cups	2 cups (28 g)	12	2	1	150
Pure De-lite Truffle, Amaretto Chocolate	1 truffle (12 g)	.6	0	1	61
Pure De-lite Truffle, Espresso Chocolate	1 truffle (12 g)	.9	0	.9	57
Pure De-lite Truffle, Hazelnut	1 truffle (12 g)	.9	0	.9	57
Pure De-lite Truffle, Mint	1 truffle (12 g)	.3	0	1	60
Pure De-lite Truffle, Orange	1 truffle (12 g)	.3	0	1	60
Pure De-lite Truffle Bar, Dark Chocolate Mint	1 bar (28 g)	13	2	1	160
Pure De-lite Truffle Bar, Milk Chocolate Caramel	1 bar (28 g)	16	2	0	140
Pure De-lite Truffle Bar, Milk Chocolate Hazelnut	1 bar (28 g)	12	2	1	160
Pure De-lite Truffle Bar, Milk Chocolate Peanut Butter	1 bar (28 g)	13	2	1	160
Pure De-lite Truffle, Peanut Butter	1 truffle (12 g)	1.4	1.4	0	62

60 CANDY

FOOD	SERVING	TOTAL CARBS (G)	NET CARBS (G)	FIBER (G)	CALORIES
Pure De-lite White Chocolate Bar	1 bar (38 g)	22	4	0	190
Russell Stover Low Carb Chocolate Wafers	2 pieces	15.8	1.6	.7	130
Russell Stover Low Carb Chocolate Covered Peanuts	25 pieces	16.5	3	2.1	210
Russell Stover Low Carb Chocolate Mousse Medallions	2 pieces	28.2	.5	.5	120
Russell Stover Low Carb French Mint	5 pieces	22	1	.9	100
Russell Stover Low Carb Milk Chocolate & Almonds	5 pieces	21	1	1.3	200
Russell Stover Low Carb Milk Chocolate & Almond Miniatures	2 pieces	12.2	.6	.7	110
Russell Stover Low Carb Milk Chocolate Miniatures	5 pieces	22.4	1	1	190
Russell Stover Low Carb Mint Patties (3.5 oz)	3 pieces	28.7	.4	1.2	200
Russell Stover Low Carb Mint Patties (1 oz)	2 pieces	18.7	.3	.8	130
Russell Stover Low Carb Peanut Butter Crunch	4 pieces	29.4	1.1	.9	180

FOOD	SERVING	TOTAL CARBS (G)	NET CARBS (G)	FIBER (G)	CALORIES
Russell Stover Low Carb Peanut Butter Cups	4 cups	17.8	1.9	2	180
Russell Stover Low Carb Peanut Butter Medallions	2 pieces	14.5	1.4	1	130
Russell Stover Low Carb Pecan Delights (3.5 oz)	4 pieces	24	.8	2.1	180
Russell Stover Low Carb Pecan Delights (1 oz)	2 pieces	16.2	1	2	130
Russell Stover Low Carb Solid Milk Chocolate	5 pieces	22.4	1	.9	190
Russell Stover Low Carb Solid Dark Chocolate Medallions	2 pieces	12	.5	1.3	130
Russell Stover Low Carb Solid Milk Chocolate Medallions	2 pieces	13	.6	.5	110
Russell Stover Low Carb Toffee Squares (3.5 oz)	3 pieces	26	.7	.7	180
Russell Stover Low Carb Toffee Squares (1 oz)	2 pieces	16.1	.4	0	110
Russell Stover Low Carb Truffle Cups	4 pieces	22.8	.6	1	170

62 CANDY

FOOD	SERVING	TOTAL CARBS (G)	NET CARBS (G)	FIBER (G)	CALORIES
CANDY, LOW CARB, BY BRAND NAME					
Atkins Caramel Nut Clusters	1 serving (7 oz)	21	5	1	180
Atkins Fruit Gum	2 pieces	1.6	0	0	3
Atkins Jelly Beans	35 beans	36	4	na	120
Atkins Mints	2 mints	1.1	0	0	2
Atkins Saltwater Taffy, Assorted	6 pieces	29	0	0	110
CarboRite Chewy Fruits	19 pieces (40 g)	0	0	0	90
CarboRite Gummy Bears	17 pieces (40 g)	30	0	0	100
CarboRite Jelly Beans	26 beans (40 g)	36	3	0	100
CarboRite Sour Citrus Slices	15 pieces (40 g)	34	6	0	100
CarboRite Toffee Chews, Chocolate	4 pieces (40 g)	33	2.5	t	120
CarboRite Toffee Chews, Vanilla	4 pieces (40 g)	33	2.5	t	120
CarboRite Chocolate Covered Raisins	35 pieces (40 g)	9	7	2	180
CarboRite Chocolate Covered Almonds	9 pieces (40 g)	18	2	2	210
CarboRite Candy Coated Chocolate	1 bag (30 g)	24	1	5	120
CarboRite Candy Coated Chocolate Covered Peanuts	1 bag (35 g)	24	2.5	5	150
Gol D Lite Chocolate Raisins D Lite	1 serving (25 g)	16	6	1	115

CANDY

FOOD	SERVING	TOTAL CARBS (G)	NET CARBS (G)	FIBER (G)	CALORIES
Gol D Lite Chocolate Almonds D Lite	1 serving (25 g)	10	.5	1.5	143
Gol D Lite Chews, Fruit	1 serving (25 g)	10	0	1.5	68
Gol D Lite Chocolate Croquants D Lite	1 serving (25 g)	12.5	.1	0	113
Gol D Lite Caramel D Lite	1 serving (25 g)	16.5	.7	1.2	79
Gol D Lite Caramel Nut D Lite	1 serving (25 g)	10.5	0	1.5	54
Gol D Lite Disco Nuts	1 serving (25 g)	14.8	1.6	.7	95
Gol D Lite European Mix Lollipops	1 lollipop (10 g)	9.3	0	0	43
Gol D Lite Fruit Gums, Cola Bottles	1 serving (25 g)	19	0	0	50
Gol D Lite Fancy Fruit Gums, Apples & Pears	1 serving (25 g)	19	0	0	50
Gol D Lite Fancy Fruit Gums, Peaches	1 serving (25 g)	19	0	0	50
Gol D Lite Fruit Gums, Cherries	1 serving (25 g)	19	0	0	50
Gol D Lite Hard Candies, Coffee	1 serving (25 g)	24	0	.2	65
Gol D Lite Hard Candies, Coffee & Cream	1 serving (25 g)	24	0	.2	65
Gol D Lite Mint D Lite	1 serving (25 g)	12.8	0	1.9	50
Gol D Lite Sesame Crunch	1 serving (25 g)	21	0	.4	75
Gol D Lite Wheat Puff D Lite	1 serving (25 g)	7.8	0	3.9	77

CANDY

FOOD	SERVING	TOTAL CARBS (G)	NET CARBS (G)	FIBER (G)	CALORIES
La Nouba Chocolate Marshmallows	1 serving (15 g)	9	.3	0	47.3
La Nouba Marshmallows	1 serving (7.5 g)	5.8	0	0	15.3
Lean Protein Bites, Peanut Butter Covered Crunch	1 bag	1	1	0	120
Low Carb Success Sweet Nut'ns	¼ cup	9	2	2	150
Megan's Candied Pecans, Cinnamon	1 serving (2 oz)	8	2	6	395
Megan's Candied Pecans, Butter Rum	1 serving (2 oz)	8	3	5	400
Megan's Candied Pecans, Caramel	1 serving (2 oz)	8	3	5	400
Megan's Candied Pecans, Orange Spice	1 serving (2 oz)	8	2	6	395
Nestlé Nips, Caramel	2 pieces (14 g)	9	0	na	50
Nestlé Nips, Coffee	2 pieces (14 g)	9	0	na	50
Pure De-lite Gummy Zoo Animals	6 pieces	20	0	0	68
Russell Stover Low Carb Jelly Beans	35 pieces	36	4	9	90
Sugar Free Lollipops	2 lollipops (15 g)	15	0	0	55
Think Thin! Chocolaty Almonds	10 pieces (40 g)	16	1	2	220
Think Thin! Chocolaty Peanuts	27 pieces (40 g)	16	1	2	220
Think Thin! Gummy Bears	17 pieces (41 g)	31	0	0	90

FOOD	SERVING	TOTAL CARBS (G)	NET CARBS (G)	FIBER (G)	CALORIES
Think Thin! Gum Drops	13 pieces (42 g)	34	1	0	90
Think Thin! Jelly Beans	33 pieces (40 g)	34	0	0	80
Think Thin! Peanut T & T's	21 pieces (40 g)	21	2	2	220
Think Thin! Sour Worms	4 pieces (41 g)	31	0	0	90
Think Thin! Sour Citrus Slices	13 pieces (42 g)	33	0	0	90

CEREALS

CEREALS, COLD

FOOD	SERVING	TOTAL CARBS (G)	NET CARBS (G)	FIBER (G)	CALORIES
100% Bran Cereal (Post)	⅓ cup	22	14	8	82
All-Bran (Kellogg's)	½ cup	23	13	10	81
All-Bran Extra Fiber (Kellogg's)	½ cup	20	7	13	50
All-Bran Bran Buds (Kellogg's)	⅓ cup	24	11	13	74
Apple Cinnamon Cheerios (General Mills)	¾ cup	25	24	1	118
Apple flavored cereal	1 cup	27	26	1	117
Banana Nut Crunch (Post)	1 cup	44	40	4	249
Banana Nut Harvest (Atkins)	⅔ cup	11	5	6	100
Basic 4 (General Mills)	1 cup	42	39	3	202
Blueberry Bounty w/Almonds (Atkins)	⅔ cup	10	4	6	100
Bran Flakes (Post)	¾ cup	24	19	5	96

CEREALS

FOOD	SERVING	TOTAL CARBS (G)	NET CARBS (G)	FIBER (G)	CALORIES
Carb Well High Protein Cereal, Cinnamon Crunch (Post)	1 serving (30 g)	14	9	5	110
Carb Well High Protein Cereal, Golden Crunch (Post)	1 serving (30 g)	14	9	5	110
Chocolate-flavored crisp cereal	¾ cup	27	26	1	118
Chocolate-flavored puff cereal	1 cup	26	25	1	117
Cocoa Crisp (Keto)	⅔ cup	4	3	1	110
Cinnamon Toast w/Flaxseed & Nuts (Gram's Gourmet)	⅓ cup	7	3	4	234
Complete Oat Bran Flakes (Kellogg's)	¾ cup	23	19	4	105
Complete Wheat Bran Flakes (Kellogg's)	¾ cup	23	18	5	92
Cookie crisp–type cereal	1 cup	26	26	t	117
Corn-based puff cereal	1 cup	28	28	t	118
Cracklin' Oat Bran (Kellogg's)	¾ cup	39	33	6	225
Cranberry Nut (Protein Crunch)	⅓ cup	7	2	2	160
Crisp Original (Keto)	⅔ cup	3	3	0	110
Crunchy Almond Crisp (Atkins)	⅔ cup	8	3	5	100
Crunchy Bran (Quaker)	¾ cup	23	18	5	90

FOOD	SERVING	TOTAL CARBS (G)	NET CARBS (G)	FIBER (G)	CALORIES
Fiber One (General Mills)	½ cup	24	10	14	59
Frosted flakes	¾ cup	28	27	1	114
Frosted Flakes, Apple Cinnamon (Keto)	¾ cup	9	3	1	110
Frosted Flakes, Classic (Keto)	¾ cup	9	3	1	110
Frosted Flakes, Honey Nut (Keto)	¾ cup	9	3	2	110
Frosted rice crisp cereal	¾ cup	27	27	t	114
Frosted wheat flake cereal	¾ cup	27	26	1	112
Fruit & Fibre (Post)	1 cup	42	37	5	212
Fruit-flavored cereal	1 cup	26	26	1	118
Graham cracker cereal	¾ cup	25	25	1	112
Granola, Apple Cinnamon (MiniCarb)	½ cup	29	4	25	285
Granola, Cinnamon Nutrageous (Flax-O-Meal)	½ cup	15	1	4	210
Granola, Cranberry Macrageous (Flax-O-Meal)	½ cup	13	2	4	190
Granola, Wild Cherry Nutrageous (Flax-O-Meal)	½ cup	16	2	4	210
Granola, plain	1 cup	79	72	7	499
Granola w/Raisins	1 cup	76	70	6	468
Granola w/Raisins, Low Fat (Kellogg's)	⅔ cup	48	45	3	231

CEREALS

FOOD	SERVING	TOTAL CARBS (G)	NET CARBS (G)	FIBER (G)	CALORIES
Granola w/o Raisins, Low Fat (Kellogg's)	½ cup	39	36	3	186
Granola w/Raisins, Low Fat (Quaker)	½ cup	41	24	17	195
Grape-Nuts (Post)	½ cup	47	42	5	208
Grape-Nuts Flakes (Post)	¾ cup	24	19	3	106
Great Grains (Post)	⅔ cup	40	36	4	204
Hi-Lo, High Protein, Low Sugar Cereal (Nutritious Living)	½ cup	11	5	6	90
Hi-Lo, High Protein, Low Sugar Cereal w/Strawberries (Nutritious Living)	½ cup	11	5	6	90
Honey nut flavored cereal	1 cup	46	43	3	214
Honey roasted oat cereal	¾ cup	25	23	2	118
Kashi GoLean (Kellogg's)	50 g	35	22.5	12.5	157
Kashi GoLean Crunch! (Kellogg's)	50 g	34	26.5	7.5	188
Kashi Good Friends (Kellogg's)	50 g	40	26.5	13.5	154
Kashi Heart to Heart (Kellogg's)	50 g	38	30.5	7.5	178
Life (Quaker)	¾ cup	25	23	2	120
Maple & Brown Sugar w/Flaxseed & Nuts (Gram's Gourmet)	⅓ cup	7	3	4	234

CEREALS

FOOD	SERVING	TOTAL CARBS (G)	NET CARBS (G)	FIBER (G)	CALORIES
Multi-Bran Chex (General Mills)	1 cup	41	35	6	166
MultiGrain Cheerios (General Mills)	1 cup	24	21	3	108
Mueslix (Kellogg's)	⅔ cup	40	36	4	198
Nutlettes Cereal (Dixie Diners' Club)	1 pkt (45 g)	12	4	8	133
Oat, corn, puffed	1⅓ cups	26	25	1	115
Oat, corn, puffed mixture, presweetened, w/marshmallows	1 cup	25	25	0	115
Oat, corn, & wheat squares, maple flavored	1 cup	24	23	1	129
Oatmeal crisp w/almonds cereal	1 cup	42	38	4	218
Oatmeal crisp w/apples cereal	1 cup	45	41	4	207
Oreo O's (Post)	¾ cup	22	20	2	112
Peanut butter crunch cereal	1 cup	28	27	1	150
Protein Crunch (Protein Crunch)	⅓ cup	5	4	1	150
Protein Crunch, No Sugar Added (Protein Crunch)	⅓ cup	3	2	1	150
Puffed rice, presweetened	¾ cup	24	24	0	108
Puffed wheat, presweetened, fruit flavored	¾ cup	25	25	0	107

CEREALS

FOOD	SERVING	TOTAL CARBS (G)	NET CARBS (G)	FIBER (G)	CALORIES
Raisin Bran (Kellogg's)	1 cup	45	38	7	188
Raisin Bran (Post)	1 cup	46	38	8	187
Raisin Nut Bran (General Mills)	1 cup	41	36	5	209
Rice Chex (General Mills)	1¼ cup	27	27	t	117
Shredded Wheat (Post)	2 biscuits	38	33	5	156
Shredded Wheat, Spoon Sized (Post)	1 cup	41	35	6	167
Shredded Wheat 'N Bran (Post)	1¼ cups	47	39	8	197
Smaps, Sweet Maple Flavor Cereal (Dixie Diners' Club)	½ cup (28 g)	9	2	7	71
Smart Start (Kellogg's)	1 cup	43	41	2	182
Special K (Kellogg's)	1 cup	22	22	t	117
Total, Corn Flakes (General Mills)	1½ cups	26	26	t	112
Total, Raisin Bran (General Mills)	1 cup	41	38	5	171
Total, Whole Grain (General Mills)	¾ cup	22	20	2	97
Uncle Sam Cereal (U.S. Mills)	1 cup	36	25	11	237
Vanilla Almond Crunch w/Flaxseed & Nuts (Gram's Gourmet)	⅓ cup	7	3	4	234
Waffle crisp cereal	1 cup	24	23.5	.5	129
Wheaties (General Mills)	1 cup	24	21	3	107

CEREALS

FOOD	SERVING	TOTAL CARBS (G)	NET CARBS (G)	FIBER (G)	CALORIES
CEREALS, HOT					
Apple Cinnamon (Atkins)	1 pouch	8	3	5	70
Apple Cinnamon & Spice (Atkins)	1 pouch	8	3	5	90
Apple Cinnamon (Keto)	2 scoops (40 g)	12	3	9	150
Banana Nut (Keto)	2 scoops (40 g)	12	3	9	150
Blueberry & Creme (Keto)	2 scoops (40 g)	14	5	9	160
Blueberry & Creme (Keto)	1 pkt (39 g)	14	5	9	160
Country Spice, Instant (CarbSense)	½ cup (40 g)	15	3	12	130
Corn grits, instant, cheddar cheese flavor, prepared w/water	1 pkt	20	19	1	99
Corn grits, white, w/o salt	½ cup	16	16	t	73
Corn grits, yellow, w/o salt	½ cup	16	16	t	73
Corn Grits, Instant, Butter Flavor (Quaker)	1 pkt	21	20	1	101
Corn Grits, Instant, Cheddar Cheese Flavor (Quaker)	1 pkt	20	20	1	99
Corn Grits, Instant, Plain (Quaker)	1 pkt	21	20	1	89
Cream of Flax, Cinnamon Toast (Gram's Gourmet)	½ cup (40 g)	11	3	8	142

72 CEREALS

FOOD	SERVING	TOTAL CARBS (G)	NET CARBS (G)	FIBER (G)	CALORIES
Cream of Flax, Maple & Brown Sugar (Gram's Gourmet)	½ cup (40 g)	11	3	8	142
Cream of Flax, Vanilla Almond (Gram's Gourmet)	½ cup (40 g)	11	3	8	142
Cream of Rice, w/o salt (Kraft)	½ cup	14	14	t	63
Cream of Wheat, Instant, w/o salt (Kraft)	½ cup	16	15	1	77
Cream of Wheat, Mix 'n Eat, Plain (Kraft)	1 pkt	21	21	t	102
Cream of Wheat, Quick, w/o salt (Kraft)	½ cup	13	12	1	64
Cream of Wheat, Regular, w/o salt (Kraft)	½ cup	14	13	1	66
Farina, w/o salt	½ cup	12	10	2	58
Flax-O-Meal, Butter Pecan (Low Carb Success)	½ cup	12	2	10	149
Flax-O-Meal, Cinnamon & Spice (Low Carb Success)	½ cup	13	1	12	130
Flax-O-Meal, Strawberries & Cream (Low Carb Success)	½ cup	14	2	12	132
Flax-O-Meal, Vanilla Almond (Low Carb Success)	½ cup	12	2	10	143

CEREALS 73

FOOD	SERVING	TOTAL CARBS (G)	NET CARBS (G)	FIBER (G)	CALORIES
Malt-O-Meal, Plain, w/o salt	½ cup	13	12.5	.5	61
Maypo, w/o salt	¾ cup	24	20	4	128
Milk Chocolate, Flaxseed/Wheat Bran (MiniCarb)	½ cup (40 g)	17	4	13	140
Multigrain oatmeal, dry	½ cup	29	26.5	2.5	133
Natural Cereal (Atkins)	1 pkt	8	3	5	90
Nestum (Nestlé)	½ cup	17	13.5	3.5	95
Oat bran	½ cup	25	19	6	146
Oatmeal, instant, w/apples & cinnamon, prepared w/water	1 pkt	26	25	1	125
Oatmeal, instant, w/cinnamon & spice, prepared w/water	1 pkt	35	32	3	177
Oatmeal, instant, w/maple & brown sugar, prepared w/water	1 pkt	31	29	3	153
Oatmeal, instant, w/raisins & spice, prepared w/water	1 pkt	32	30	2	161
Oatmeal, microwave, apple spice	1 pkt	35	32	3	166
Oatmeal, microwave, brown sugar & cinnamon	1 pkt	31	28	3	155
Oatmeal, microwave, cinnamon & double raisin	1 pkt	35	32	3	169

CEREALS

FOOD	SERVING	TOTAL CARBS (G)	NET CARBS (G)	FIBER (G)	CALORIES
Oatmeal, Quick 'n Hearty, Regular Flavor (Quaker)	1 pkt	19	16.5	2.5	106
Oats, instant, plain	½ cup	12	10	2	69
Oats, instant, w/bran & raisins	1 pkt	30	24	6	158
Oats, old fashioned, w/o salt	½ cup	27	23	4	150
Old Fashioned Oatmeal (Keto)	2 scoops (40 g)	14	5	9	160
Old Fashioned Oatmeal (Keto)	1 pkt (39 g)	14	5	9	160
Peaches & Cream (Atkins)	1 pouch	8	3	5	90
Ralston 100% Wheat Hot Cereal	½ cup	14	11	3	67
Roasted Hazelnut, Instant (CarbSense)	½ cup (40 g)	15	3	12	140
Roman Meal Hot Cereal, Original w/Oats	½ cup	17	13	4	85
Strawberry & Creme (Keto)	2 scoops (40 g)	14	5	9	160
Sweet Maple (Atkins)	1 pouch	8	3	5	90
Wheatena	½ cup	14	11	3	68
Whole wheat, hot natural cereal	½ cup	17	15	2	75

CHEESE

CHEESE, FULL FAT

FOOD	SERVING	TOTAL CARBS (G)	NET CARBS (G)	FIBER (G)	CALORIES
Blue	1 oz	1	1	0	100
Brick	1 oz	1	1	0	105
Brie	1 oz	t	t	0	95
Camembert	1 oz	t	t	0	85
Caraway	1 oz	1	1	0	107
Cheddar	1 oz	t	t	0	114
Colby	1 oz	1	1	0	112
Cream	1 tbsp	0	0	0	51
Creamed cottage, large or small curd, full fat	½ cup, small curd, not packed	3	3	0	116
Creamed Cottage, full fat w/fruit	½ cup, not packed	15	15	0	140
Edam	1 oz	t	t	0	101
Feta	1 oz	1	1	0	75
Fontina	1 oz	t	t	0	110
Goat, hard type	1 oz	1	1	0	128
Goat, semisoft type	1 oz	1	1	0	103
Goat, soft type	1 oz	t	t	0	76
Gouda	1 oz	1	1	0	101
Gruyère	1 oz	t	t	0	117
Limburger	1 oz	t	t	0	93
Low sodium, cheddar or Colby	1 oz	1	1	0	113
Monterey	1 oz	t	t	0	106
Mozzarella, whole milk	1 oz	1	1	0	80

76 CHEESE

FOOD	SERVING	TOTAL CARBS (G)	NET CARBS (G)	FIBER (G)	CALORIES
Mozzarella, whole milk, low moisture	1 oz	1	1	0	90
Muenster	1 oz	t	t	0	104
Neufchâtel	1 oz	1	1	0	74
Parmesan, grated	2 tbsp	t	t	0	46
Parmesan, hard	1 oz	1	1	0	111
Port de Salut	1 oz	t	t	0	100
Provolone	1 oz	1	1	0	100
Ricotta, whole milk	½ cup	4	4	0	214
Romano	1 oz	1	1	0	110
Roquefort	1 oz	1	1	0	105
Swiss	1 oz	1	1	0	107
CHEESES, REDUCED FAT					
Cheddar, low fat	1 oz	1	1	0	98
Colby, low fat	1 oz	1	1	0	98
Cottage, low fat, 1% milkfat	½ cup	3	3	0	81
Cottage, low fat, 2% milkfat	½ cup	4	4	0	102
Cottage, non fat	½ cup	1	1	0	62
Mozzarella, part skim milk	1 oz	1	1	0	72
Mozzarella, part skim milk, low moisture	1 oz	1	1	0	79
Ricotta, part skim	½ cup	6	6	0	170
CHEESE, PROCESSED					
American, processed, pasteurized, w/o disodium phosphate	1 oz	t	t	0	106

FOOD	SERVING	TOTAL CARBS (G)	NET CARBS (G)	FIBER (G)	CALORIES
American, processed, pasteurized, w/ disodium phosphate	1 oz	t	t	0	106
American spread, w/o disodium phosphate	1 oz	2	2	0	82
American spread, w/ disodium phosphate	1 oz	2	2	0	82
Cheddar, processed, pasteurized, low sodium	1 slice	0	0	0	79
Cheese spread	1 oz	3	3	0	85
Cheese sauce	2 tbsp	3	3	t	91
Imitation cheese, American or cheddar, low cholesterol	1 cubic inch	0	0	0	70
Pimento processed cheese	1 oz	t	t	0	106
Swiss processed cheese	1 oz	t	t	0	95

COFFEE AND TEA

COFFEE

FOOD	SERVING	TOTAL CARBS (G)	NET CARBS (G)	FIBER (G)	CALORIES
Brewed	1 cup	t	t	0	5
Brewed, decaf	1 cup	t	t	0	5
Cafe Francais flavored coffee, powdered (Kraft)	1 serving	7	7	t	62
Cappuccino flavored coffee, powdered w/sugar	2 rounded tsp	11	11	0	62
Cappuccino Flavored Coffee (Atkins)	1 bottle (9.5 fl oz)	5	5	0	120

COFFEE AND TEA

FOOD	SERVING	TOTAL CARBS (G)	NET CARBS (G)	FIBER (G)	CALORIES
Cappuccino Flavored Coffee, Sugar Free (Atkins)	3 tbsp	3	3	0	50
Chicory added, instant	1 cup	2	2	0	10
Espresso, restaurant prepared	100 g	1.5	1.5	0	9
French flavor coffee, powder	2 rounded tsp	6	6	0	57
French vanilla café flavored coffee, powder	1 serving	10	10	t	65
French vanilla flavor, sugar free, fat free, instant, prepared	1 cup	5	5	t	25
French mocha flavor, sugar free, fat free, instant, prepared	1 cup	5	4	1	24
Hazelnut Crème Coffee Drink (Achiev One)	1 bottle (9.5 fl oz)	5	5	0	120
Instant	1 cup	t	t	0	5
Instant, decaf	1 cup	t	t	0	4
Mocha Java Coffee Drink (Achiev One)	1 bottle (9.5 fl oz)	5	5	0	120
Mocha flavored coffee, powder	2 rounded tsp	8	8	t	51
Suisse Mocha flavored coffee, powder (Kraft)	1 serving	9	9	t	57
Vanilla Nut Coffee Drink (Achiev One)	1 bottle (9.5 fl oz)	5	5	0	120

FOOD	SERVING	TOTAL CARBS (G)	NET CARBS (G)	FIBER (G)	CALORIES
TEA					
Brewed	1 cup	t	t	0	2
Brewed, decaf	1 cup	1	1	0	2
Chai Black Tea Latte, Spiced, Instant (Da Vinci)	1.5 tbsp	0	0	0	0
Chamomile, brewed	1 cup	t	t	0	2
Decaffeinated Tea, Sweetened, Instant, No Sugar (Carb Options)	1 cup	0	0	0	0
Green Tea w/Orange Passionfruit Twist, Instant, Sweetened, No Sugar (Carb Options)	1 cup	0	0	0	0
Green Tea Concentrate w/Yerba Maté, Instant (Da Vinci)	2 tbsp	0	0	0	0
Herbal, brewed	1 cup	t	t	0	2
Instant, unsweetened	1 cup	t	t	0	2
Instant, Sugar Free Lemon Flavored Tea Blend (Atkins)	1 cup	0	0	0	0
Instant, unsweetened, lemon flavored	1 cup	1	1	0	5
Lemon flavored tea, instant w/sugar	1 cup	22	22	0	88
Lemon Flavored Tea, Sweetened, Instant, No Sugar (Carb Options)	1 cup	0	0	0	0

80 CONDIMENTS AND MAYONNAISE

FOOD	SERVING	TOTAL CARBS (G)	NET CARBS (G)	FIBER (G)	CALORIES
Lemon Tea Concentrate, Instant (Da Vinci)	2 tbsp	0	0	0	0
Lemon flavored ice tea, ready to drink	1 cup	20	20	0	89
Sugar free, low calorie, w/aspartame	1 cup	t	t	0	3
Sugar free, low calorie, lemon flavored w/saccharin	1 cup	1	1	0	5

CONDIMENTS AND MAYONNAISE
CONDIMENTS

FOOD	SERVING	TOTAL CARBS (G)	NET CARBS (G)	FIBER (G)	CALORIES
A1 Steak Sauce	1 tbsp	3	3	na	15
Barbecue sauce	2 tbsp	4	4	t	23
Catsup	1 tbsp	4	4	t	16
Catsup, Green (Heinz)	1 tbsp	5	5	0	20
Catsup, low sodium	1 tbsp	4	4	t	16
Catsup, Ketch-a-Tomato (Atkins)	1 tbsp	2	1	1	10
Catsup, Low Calorie (Carb Options)	1 tbsp	t	t	0	5
Catsup, Ketchup (Keto)	1 tbsp	1	1	0	5
Catsup, Tomato Ketchup (Walden Farms)	2 tbsp	0	0	0	0
Catsup, Rocky Mountain Ketchup (Steel's)	1 tbsp	0	0	0	10
Chili Sauce (Chef Mate Hot Dog, Nestlé)	1 tbsp	2	2	t	17

CONDIMENTS AND MAYONNAISE

FOOD	SERVING	TOTAL CARBS (G)	NET CARBS (G)	FIBER (G)	CALORIES
Cocktail Sauce (Del Monte)	2 tbsp	12	12	na	50
Enchilada Sauce (Ortega)	2 tbsp	1	1	t	15
Horseradish	1 tbsp	2	2	t	7
Hot pepper sauce	¼ tsp	t	t	0	0
Mustard (Grey Poupon)	1 tbsp	0	0	na	15
Mustard, yellow	1 tbsp	1	1	t	10
Picante Sauce (Ortega)	2 tbsp	2	2	0	10
Picante Sauce, Medium (La Victoria)	2 tbsp	1	1	t	8
Picante Sauce, Mild (La Victoria)	2 tbsp	1	1	t	8
Salsa	2 tbsp	2	2	t	9
Salsa, black bean & corn	2 tbsp	3	2.5	.5	16
Salsa, Chunky Chili Dip (La Victoria)	2 tbsp	2	2	t	9
Salsa, Green Chili, Mild (La Victoria)	2 tbsp	1	1	t	8
Salsa, Green Jalapeño (La Victoria)	2 tbsp	1	1	t	10
Salsa Ranchero, Hot (La Victoria)	2 tbsp	2	2	t	9
Salsa, Red Jalapeño (La Victoria)	2 tbsp	2	2	t	12
Salsa, Thick 'N Chunky, Hot (La Victoria)	2 tbsp	1	1	t	8
Salsa, Thick 'N Chunky, Medium (La Victoria)	2 tbsp	1	1	t	8

CONDIMENTS AND MAYONNAISE

FOOD	SERVING	TOTAL CARBS (G)	NET CARBS (G)	FIBER (G)	CALORIES
Salsa, Thick 'N Chunky, Mild (La Victoria)	2 tbsp	1	1	t	8
Spaghetti/marinara sauce	½ cup	10	8	2	71
Tabasco sauce	1 tsp	t	t	0	1
Taco Sauce, Green, Mild (La Victoria)	2 tbsp	2	2	t	9
Taco Sauce, Red, Medium (La Victoria)	2 tbsp	3	3	t	13
Taco Sauce, Red, Mild (La Victoria)	2 tbsp	3	3	t	13
Tartar sauce, low calorie	1 tbsp	2	2	na	31
Teriyaki sauce, generic	2 tbsp	6	6	0	30
Teriyaki Marinade & Sauce (Kikkoman)	2 tbsp	4	4	0	30
Teriyaki Sauce (Nestlé)	2 tbsp	7	7	0	42
Vinegar	1 tbsp	t	t	0	1
Worcestershire sauce	1 tsp	0	0	0	0
MAYONNAISE					
Mayonnaise, regular	1 tbsp	4	4	0	57
Mayonnaise, regular, soybean based	1 tbsp	t	t	0	99
Mayonnaise, Fat Free (Kraft)	2 tbsp	4	4	t	22
Mayonnaise, made w/tofu	2 tbsp	2	2	0	96
Mayonnaise, imitation, milk cream	2 tbsp	4	4	0	30
Mayonnaise, imitation, soybean based	2 tbsp	5	5	0	70

FOOD	SERVING	TOTAL CARBS (G)	NET CARBS (G)	FIBER (G)	CALORIES
Mayonnaise, imitation, soybean based, w/o cholesterol	1 tbsp	2	2	0	68
Mayonnaise, Light (Kraft)	2 tbsp	3	3	0	100
Miracle Whip, Light (Kraft)	2 tbsp	5	5	0	74
Miracle Whip Free, Nonfat (Kraft)	2 tbsp	5	5	t	27
Whipped Dressing (Carb Options)	1 tbsp	0	0	0	50

COOKIES AND BROWNIES

BROWNIES

FOOD	SERVING	TOTAL CARBS (G)	NET CARBS (G)	FIBER (G)	CALORIES
Brownies, prepared from recipe	1 brownie (2" x 2")	12	12	na	112
Brownies, commercially prepared	1 package, twin wrapped	39	38	1	247
Brownies, commercially prepared	1 brownie, large (2¾" x ⅞")	36	35	1	227
Brownies, Sugar Free, Pecan/Walnut (Joseph's)	9 brownies (26 g)	15	2	1	150
Brownie Mix, Chocolate Fudge (Keto)	1 brownie	2	1	1	59
Brownie Mix, Fudge Brownie (Keto)	1 brownie (2" x 2")	9	2	5	70
Brownie Mix, w/Almonds (Dixie Diners' Club)	1 brownie (2" x 2")	1	1	0	165

84 COOKIES AND BROWNIES

FOOD	SERVING	TOTAL CARBS (G)	NET CARBS (G)	FIBER (G)	CALORIES
Brownie Mix, Fudge Brownie (Dixie Diners' Club)	1 serving (0.5 oz)	2	1	1	31
Brownie Mix, Brownie & Cake Mix (Pure De-lite)	1 brownie (22 g)	4	2	1	50
Brownie mix, Chocolate (MiniCarb)	1 brownie (40 g)	10	3	8	220
COOKIES					
Almond Cookies, Sugar Free (Joseph's)	4 cookies (26 g)	13	7	0	100
Almond Cookies, Small Snack Size, Sugar Free (Joseph's)	1 bag (42 g)	19	9	1	150
Almond Cookies (Soybite)	1½ cookies (30 g)	9	1	2	170
Animal crackers	1 arrowroot biscuit	4	4	t	22
Apricot filled cookies	1 serving	16	16	t	100
Banana Cookies (Soybite)	1½ cookies (30 g)	9	1	2	170
Brownie Cookies, Soy Fudgies (Glenny's)	3 cookies	14	3	1	70
Butter cookies, commercially prepared, unenriched	1 cookie	3	3	0	23
Butter cookies, commercially prepared, enriched	1 cookie	3	3	0	23
Chocolate chip cookie, refrigerated dough	1 serving	18	17	1	127

COOKIES AND BROWNIES 85

FOOD	SERVING	TOTAL CARBS (G)	NET CARBS (G)	FIBER (G)	CALORIES
Chocolate chip cookie, refrigerated dough, baked	1 cookie, medium (2¼" dia)	8	8	t	59
Chocolate chip cookie, prepared from recipe, made w/margarine	1 cookie, medium (2¼" dia)	9	9	t	78
Chocolate chip cookie, prepared from recipe, made w/margarine	1 bar (2" x 2")	19	18	1	156
Chocolate chip cookie, prepared from recipe, made w/butter	1 cookie, medium (2¼" dia)	9	8	1	78
Chocolate chip cookie, commercially prepared, soft type	1 cookie	9	9	t	69
Chocolate Chip Cookies (CarboRite)	1 cookie (30 g)	12	2	4	120
Chocolate Chip Cookies (Joseph's)	4 cookies (26 g)	13	7	0	100
Chocolate Chip Cookies (Soybite)	1½ cookies (30 g)	9	1	2	170
Chocolate Cookies (Soybite)	1½ cookies (30 g)	9	1	2	170
Chocolate Chip Cookies (Low Carb Creations)	1 cookie	10	2	2	166
Chocolate Chip, Low Carb Cookies (Super Chip)	2 cookies (27 g)	10	0	3	100
Chocolate Covered Wafers, Lite Rafts (Gol D Lite)	1 serving (10.5 g)	5.5	0.5	0	45

86 COOKIES AND BROWNIES

FOOD	SERVING	TOTAL CARBS (G)	NET CARBS (G)	FIBER (G)	CALORIES
Chocolate Fudge Cookie (Pure De-lite)	1 cookie (62 g)	29	0	5	210
Chocolate Raspberry Cookies, Soy Fudgies (Glenny's)	3 cookies	14	3	1	70
Chocolate Walnut, Sugar Free (Joseph's)	4 cookies (26 g)	14	4	0	100
Chocolate Walnut, Sugar Free, Small Snack Size (Joseph's)	1 bag (42 g)	20	8	1	150
Chocolate sandwich cookie w/extra crème filling	1 cookie	9	9	t	65
Chocolate sandwich cookie w/crème filling, regular, chocolate-coated	1 cookie	11	10	1	82
Chocolate sandwich cookie w/ crème filling	1 cookie	7	7	t	47
Chocolate wafers	1 wafer	4	4	t	26
Cinnamon Cookies (Soybite)	1½ cookies (30 g)	9	1	2	170
Coconut Cookies (Soybite)	1½ cookies (30 g)	9	1	2	170
Coconut, Sugar Free (Joseph's)	4 cookies (26 g)	14	4	0	105
Coconut, Small, Sugar Free (Joseph's)	1 bag (42 g)	21	11	1	150
Coconut Cookies (Low Carb Creations)	1 cookie	6	2	1	135

COOKIES AND BROWNIES 87

FOOD	SERVING	TOTAL CARBS (G)	NET CARBS (G)	FIBER (G)	CALORIES
Coconut macaroons, prepared from recipe	1 cookie, medium (2" dia)	17	17	t	97
Coffee Cookies (Soybite)	1½ cookies (30 g)	9	1	2	170
Cookie Cremes, Chocolate (CarbRite)	3 cookies (42 g)	23	3	2	170
Cookie Cremes, Vanilla (CarboRite)	3 cookies (42 g)	23	3	2	180
Cookie Crisp (Gol D Lite)	1 serving (10.5 g)	6.5	3.8	.2	50
Crisp Wafers (CarboRite)	1 bar (0.9 g)	14	1	1	120
Fig bars	1 cookie	11	10	1	56
Fortune cookie	1 cookie	7	7	t	30
Frosted Island Coconut (Low Carb Enchantments)	1 cookie (28 g)	11	2	1	130
Frosted Zesty Lemon (Low Carb Enchantments)	1 cookie (28 g)	11	2	1	120
Fudge Covered Grahams (Nabisco SnackWell's CarbWell Cookies)	1 cookie (27 g)	18	17	1	120
Fudge Striped Shortbread (Nabisco SnackWell's CarbWell Cookies)	1 cookie (24 g)	16	15	1	110
Fudge, cake type	1 cookie	16	15	1	73
Gingersnaps	1 cookie	5	5	t	29

COOKIES AND BROWNIES

FOOD	SERVING	TOTAL CARBS (G)	NET CARBS (G)	FIBER (G)	CALORIES
Gingersnaps	1 large (3½" to 4" dia)	25	24	1	133
Gourmet Cookies, Chocolate Chip (Atkins)	1 cookie	11	2	1	140
Gourmet Cookies, Peanut Butter (Atkins)	1 cookie	9	2	1	140
Classic Chocolate Chip (Low Carb Enchantments)	1 cookie (28 g)	11	2	3	130
Graham crackers, plain or honey (includes cinnamon)	1 cracker (2½" x 2½")	5	5	t	30
Graham crackers, plain or honey (includes cinnamon)	1 large rectangular piece, 2 squares, or 4 small rectangular pieces	11	11	t	59
Graham crackers, chocolate-coated	1 cracker (2½" x 2")	9	9	t	68
Italian Style Biscotti, Chocolate (Keto)	1 cookie (28 g)	6	4	2	160
Italian Style Biscotti, Lemon Nut (Keto)	1 cookie (28 g)	6	4	2	160
Italian Style Biscotti, Vanilla Nut (Keto)	1 cookie (28 g)	6	4	2	160
Lemon Cookies, Sugar Free (Joseph's)	1 bag (42 g)	22	12	1	140
Lemon Cookies, Sugar Free, Snack Size (Joseph's)	4 cookie servings/bag (26 g)	15	9	0	95

FOOD	SERVING	TOTAL CARBS (G)	NET CARBS (G)	FIBER (G)	CALORIES
Lemon Cookies (Low Carb Creations)	1 cookie	6	2	1	137
Lemon Cookies (Soybite)	1½ cookies (30 g)	9	1	2	170
Lemon drop cookies	1 serving	15	15	t	93
Lemon snaps	1 serving	20	20	t	152
Marshmallow pies	1 pie (3" dia x ¾")	26	25	1	164
Meringue Cookies, Cappuccino (Heavenly Desserts)	1 cookie (1.5 g)	1	0	0	4
Meringue Cookies, Chocolate (Heavenly Desserts)	1 cookie (1.5 g)	1	0	0	4
Meringue Cookies, Chocolate (Atkins)	1 cookie	1	0	0	4
Meringue Cookies, Lemon (Heavenly Desserts)	1 cookie (1.5 g)	1	0	0	4
Meringue Cookies, Strawberry (Heavenly Desserts)	1 cookie (1.5 g)	1	0	0	4
Meringue Cookies, Strawberry (Atkins)	1 cookie	1	0	0	4
Meringue Cookies, Vanilla (Atkins)	1 cookie	1	0	0	4
Meringue Cookies, Vanilla (Heavenly Desserts)	1 cookie (1.5 g)	1	0	0	4
Meringue Cookies, White Chocolate (Atkins)	1 cookie	1	0	0	4

90 COOKIES AND BROWNIES

FOOD	SERVING	TOTAL CARBS (G)	NET CARBS (G)	FIBER (G)	CALORIES
Mint crème cookies	1 serving	19	19	t	108
Mint Chocolate Cookies (Low Carb Enchantments)	1 cookie (28 g)	10	3	2	130
Molasses cookies	1 medium	11	11	t	65
Molasses cookies	1 large (3½"–4" dia)	24	24	t	138
Molasses iced cookies	1 serving	20	20	t	114
Oatmeal cookies	1 serving	17	16	1	111
Oatmeal cookies, apple filled	1 serving	16	15	1	103
Oatmeal cookies, refrigerated dough, baked	1 cookie	8	8	t	39
Oatmeal cookies, prepared from recipe, w/o raisins	1 cookie (2⅝" dia)	10	10	na	90
Oatmeal cookies, prepared from recipe, w/raisins	1 cookie (2⅝" dia)	10	10	na	81
Oatmeal cookies, commercially prepared, soft type	1 cookie	10	10	t	52
Oatmeal cookies, commercially prepared, regular	1 cookie, large	12	11	1	69
Oatmeal cookies, commercially prepared, regular	1 cookie, big (3½"–4" dia)	17	16	1	96
Oatmeal Cookies, Sugar Free (Joseph's)	4 cookie/bag (26 g)	15	9	0	100

COOKIES AND BROWNIES

FOOD	SERVING	TOTAL CARBS (G)	NET CARBS (G)	FIBER (G)	CALORIES
Oatmeal Cookies, Sugar Free, Snack Size (Joseph's)	1 bag (42 g)	22	12	1	150
Oatmeal Cookies (Granny Oats)	4 cookies	10	4	3	98
Oatmeal raisin cookie	1 serving	17	16	1	98
Oatmeal iced cookie	1 serving	18	17	1	92
Peanut butter cookie	1 serving	12	11	1	85
Peanut butter cookie, refrigerated dough, baked	1 cookie	7	7	t	52
Peanut butter cookie, commercially prepared, regular	1 cookie	9	9	t	62
Peanut butter cookie, commercially prepared, soft type	1 cookie	9	9	t	50
Peanut Butter Cookie (CarboRite)	1 cookie (30 g)	12	2	4	120
Peanut Butter Cookies, Sugar Free (Joseph's)	4 cookie/bag (26 g)	13	7	0	95
Peanut Butter Cookies, Sugar Free, Snack Size (Joseph's)	1 bag (42 g)	19.5	9.5	1	140
Peanut Butter Cookies (Soybite)	1½ cookies (30 g)	9	1	2	170
Peanut Butter Cookies (Low Carb Creations)	1 cookie	7	2	2	150
Peanut Butter & Chocolate Chip Cookies (Low Carb Creations)	1 cookie	10	2	2	177

COOKIES AND BROWNIES

FOOD	SERVING	TOTAL CARBS (G)	NET CARBS (G)	FIBER (G)	CALORIES
Peanut Butter Chocolate Chunk (Low Carb Enchantments)	1 cookie (28 g)	10	3	1	130
Peanut Butter Crunch Cookie (Pure De-lite)	1 cookie (62 g)	28	0	5	210
Peanut butter sandwich cookie	1 cookie	9	9	t	52
Pecan Chip, Mini Cookie (Andre's Carbosave)	1 cookie (1 oz)	13	2	1	130
Pecan Chocolate Chip Cookie, Sugar Free (Joseph's)	4 cookie/bag (26 g)	13	6	1	95
Pecan Shortbread Cookie, Sugar Free (Joseph's)	4 cookie/bag (26 g)	14	8	0	100
Raisin cookie, soft type	1 cookie	10	10	t	51
Pecan ice box cookie	1 serving	15	15	t	75
Rasberry filled cookies	1 serving	16	16	t	84
Shortbread cookie, commercially prepared, plain	1 cookie (1⅝" square)	5	5	t	36
Shortbread cookie, commercially prepared, pecan	1 cookie (2" dia)	8	8	t	76
Shortbread Cookie (CarboRite)	1 cookie (30 g)	14	2.5	5	180
Shortbread Cookie (Low Carb Chef)	1 cookie (3 g)	1	0	1	15

COOKIES AND BROWNIES

FOOD	SERVING	TOTAL CARBS (G)	NET CARBS (G)	FIBER (G)	CALORIES
Snicker Doodle (Low Carb Enchantments)	1 cookie (28 g)	9	2	1	130
Strawberry filled cookie	1 serving	16	16	t	100
Sugar cookie, refrigerated dough, baked	1 cookie, presliced cookie dough	15	15	t	111
Sugar cookie, prepared from recipe, made w/margarine	1 cookie (3" dia)	8	8	t	66
Sugar cookie, refrigerated dough, baked	1 cookie, rolled cookie dough	10	10	t	73
Sugar cookie, commercially prepared, regular	1 cookie	10	10	t	72
Sugar wafer cookie w/crème filling	1 wafer, small (2½" x ¾" x ¼")	2	2	0	18
Sugar wafer cookie w/crème filling	1 wafer, large (3½" x 1" x ½")	6	6	t	46
Vanilla sandwich cookie, w/crème filling	1 cookie, round (1¾" dia)	7	7	t	48
Vanilla sandwich cookie, w/crème filling	1 cookie, oval (3⅛" x 1¼" x ⅜")	11	11	t	72
Vanilla wafer	1 wafer	4	4	T	28
COOKIE MIXES					
Beanit Butter Cookie Mix (Dixie Diners' Club)	1 cookie	2	1	1	127
Chocolate Truffle Mix (Dixie Diners' Club)	1 piece (0.5 oz)	2	1	1	31

CREAM AND CREAMERS

FOOD	SERVING	TOTAL CARBS (G)	NET CARBS (G)	FIBER (G)	CALORIES
Coconut Macaroonies Cookie Mix (Dixie Diners' Club)	1 cookie	2	1	1	164
Chocolate Chip Cookie Mix (Atkins)	2 cookies (2")	16	6	4	70
Chocolate Chip Cookie Mix (Keto)	1 cookie (6 g)	2	1	1	35
Chocolate Chocolate Chip Cookie Mix (Dixie Diners' Club)	1 cookie	3	2	1	153
Chocolate Chocolate Chip Cookie Mix (Atkins)	2 cookies (2")	15	6	4	60
Chocolate Covered Cookie Dough (Atkins)	40 g	22	4	1	170
Lemon Burst Cookie Mix (MiniCarb)	1 cookie (1 oz)	7	2	5	110
Oatmeal Raisin Cookie Mix (Keto)	2 cookies	2	1	1	60
Snicker Doodle Cookie Mix (MiniCarb)	1 cookie (1 oz)	7	2	5	110

CREAM AND CREAMERS

FOOD	SERVING	TOTAL CARBS (G)	NET CARBS (G)	FIBER (G)	CALORIES
Coconut cream, canned	½ cup	12	19	3	284
Creamer, nondairy, w/hydrogenated vegetable oil & soy protein	1 tbsp	2	2	0	12

FOOD	SERVING	TOTAL CARBS (G)	NET CARBS (G)	FIBER (G)	CALORIES
Creamer, nondairy, w/lauric acid oil & sodium caseinate	1 tbsp	2	2	0	12
Half-and-Half	1 tbsp	1	1	0	6
Liquid, coffee or table	1 tbsp	1	1	0	6
Whipping, heavy	1 tbsp	t	t	0	6
Sour cream	1 tbsp	1	1	0	6

DIET AND NUTRITIONAL BARS, CEREAL BARS

BARS

FOOD	SERVING	TOTAL CARBS (G)	NET CARBS (G)	FIBER (G)	CALORIES
Aramana Soy Energy Bar, Blueberry Crisp	1 bar (56 g)	33	4	6	220
Aramana Soy Energy Bar, Chocolate Crisp	1 bar (56 g)	22	3	3	220
Aramana Soy Energy Bar, Mocha Cappuccino Crisp	1 bar (56 g)	31	4	5	230
Aramana Soy Energy Bar, Peanut Butter Crisp	1 bar (56 g)	24	4	4	225
Atkins Advantage Bar, Almond Brownie	1 bar (60 g)	21	2	7	220
Atkins Advantage Bar, Chocolate Coconut	1 bar (60 g)	21	2	9	230
Atkins Advantage Bar, Chocolate Decadence	1 bar (60 g)	25	2	11	220
Atkins Advantage Bar, Chocolate Mocha Crunch	1 bar (60 g)	22	3	10	220

DIET AND NUTRITIONAL BARS, CEREAL BARS

FOOD	SERVING	TOTAL CARBS (G)	NET CARBS (G)	FIBER (G)	CALORIES
Atkins Advantage Bar, Chocolate Peanut Butter	1 bar (60 g)	21	2	10	240
Atkins Advantage Bar, Cookies 'N Crème	1 bar (60 g)	22	2	11	220
Atkins Advantage Bar, Pralines 'N Crème	1 bar (60 g)	18	3	7	250
Atkins Advantage Bar, S'mores	1 bar (60 g)	26	3	11	220
Atkins Endulge Caramel Nut Chew	1 bar (1.23 oz)	17	2	1	140
Atkins Endulge Chocolate Wafer Crisp	2 bars	15	4	3	120
Atkins Endulge Mint Wafer Crisp	2 bars	15	4	3	120
Atkins Endulge Peanut Butter Wafer Crisp	2 bars	14	4	3	120
Atkins Endulge Peanut Caramel Cluster	1 bar (35 g)	13	1	4	150
Atkins Endulge Vanilla Wafer Crisp	2 bars	15	4	3	120
Balance Bars, Chocolate	1 bar (1.7 oz)	22	21	1	200
Biochem Lo Carb Deluxe, Chocolate Mint	1 bar (72 g)	23	2	1	250
Biochem Lo Carb Deluxe, S'mores	1 bar (72 g)	21	2	1	250
Boost Bar	1 bar (1.6 oz)	29	29	t	190
Carb Options Chocolate Chip Bar	1 bar (50 g)	17	4	t	200

DIET AND NUTRITIONAL BARS, CEREAL BARS

FOOD	SERVING	TOTAL CARBS (G)	NET CARBS (G)	FIBER (G)	CALORIES
Carb Options Chocolate Peanut Butter Bar	1 bar (50 g)	17	4	t	200
Carb Options Cinnamon Delight Bar	1 bar (50 g)	17	4	0	200
CarboRite Caramel Nougat Bar	1 bar	20	0	1	100
CarboRite Chocolate Almond Bar	1 bar	14	0	1	130
CarboRite Chocolate Crisp Bar	1 bar	15	1	1	140
CarboRite Chocolate Peanut Butter Bar	1 bar	15	1	1	140
CarboRite Chocolate Truffle	1 bar	17	1	1	122
CarboRite Dark Chocolate Bar	1 bar	15	1	2	130
CarboRite Milk Chocolate Bar	1 bar	15	0	1	140
CarboRite Peanut Caramel Nougat Bar	1 bar	20	0	1	110
CarboRite Pecan Cluster Bar	1 bar	15	0	1	120
CarboRite Sugar Free Chocolate Peanut Butter Bar	1 bar	13	11	2	120
CarboRite Toffee Bar	1 bar	15	0	0	110
CarbWise Delicious Crispy Bars, Chocolate Peanut Crunch	1 bar (60 g)	23	3	t	240

DIET AND NUTRITIONAL BARS, CEREAL BARS

FOOD	SERVING	TOTAL CARBS (G)	NET CARBS (G)	FIBER (G)	CALORIES
CarbWise Delicious Crispy Bars, Chocolate Raspberry Crunch	1 bar (60 g)	24	3	t	240
CarbWise Delicious Crispy Bars, Chocolate S'mores Crunch	1 bar (60 g)	24	2	t	240
CarbWise Delicious Crispy Bars, Lemon Yogurt Crunch	1 bar (60 g)	24	4	t	240
CarbWise Gold, Rich & Creamy, Chocolate Caramel Peanut	1 bar (50 g)	18	3	0	190
Doctor's CarbRite Diet Bar, Banana Nut w/Soy Nuts	1 bar (56.7 g)	22	2	0	195
Doctor's CarbRite Diet Bar, Blueberry Cheesecake	1 bar (56.7 g)	22.5	2.5	0	199
Doctor's CarbRite Diet Bar, Chocolate Brownie	1 bar (56.7 g)	23	2.5	1	195
Doctor's CarbRite Diet Bar, Chocolate Mint Cookie	1 bar (56.7 g)	23	2.5	0	185
Doctor's CarbRite Diet Bar, Chocolate Peanut Butter	1 bar (56.7 g)	22	2.5	0	190
Doctor's CarbRite Diet Bar, Frosted Cinnamon Bun	1 bar (56.7 g)	23	2.5	1	200

DIET AND NUTRITIONAL BARS, CEREAL BARS

FOOD	SERVING	TOTAL CARBS (G)	NET CARBS (G)	FIBER (G)	CALORIES
Doctor's CarbRite Diet Bar, Raspberry Chocolate Truffle	1 bar (56.7 g)	22	2	0	195
Doctor's CarbRite Diet Bar, S'mores	1 bar (56.7 g)	22	2.5	0	188
Doctor's CarbRite Diet Bar, Toasted Coconut	1 bar (56.7 g)	24	2	1	200
Energy Bar, All Flavors (Gatorade)	1 bar (2.3 oz)	47	45.5	1.5	255
Energy, sport, or breakfast bar, generic	1 medium bar	27	25	2	202
Energy, sport, or breakfast bar, generic	1 small bar	22	18.5	3.5	140
Ensure nutrition & energy bar	1 bar (60 g)	35	34	1	230
General Mills Momentum Bar, Chocolate Caramel	1 bar (40 g)	17	3	3	150
General Mills Momentum Bar, Chocolate Peanut Butter	1 bar (40 g)	16	3	3	150
General Mills Momentum Bar, Double Chocolate	1 bar (40 g)	17	3	3	150
Hi-Lo Nutrition Bar, Chocolate Caramel	1 bar (50 g)	20	2	0	200
Hi-Lo Nutrition Bar, Chocolate Peanut	1 bar (50 g)	18	1	5	200
Hi-Lo Nutrition Bar, Peanut Butter Crisp	1 bar (30 g)	14	7	1	110

DIET AND NUTRITIONAL BARS, CEREAL BARS

FOOD	SERVING	TOTAL CARBS (G)	NET CARBS (G)	FIBER (G)	CALORIES
Keto Bar, Blueberry Cheesecake	1 bar (65 g)	21	2	4	230
Keto Bar, Caramel Nut Crunch	1 bar (56 g)	17	2	2	230
Keto Bar, Chocolate Coconut Crème	1 bar (65 g)	24	3	5	270
Keto Bar, Mini Chocolate Coconut Crème	1 bar (32 g)	12	2	2	140
Keto Bar, Chocolate Fudge	1 bar (65 g)	24	4	5	260
Keto Bar, Mini Chocolate Fudge	1 bar (32 g)	12	2	3	130
Keto Bar, Chocolate Peanut Butter	1 bar (65 g)	24	2	5	270
Keto Bar, Mini Chocolate Peanut Butter	1 bar (32 g)	12	1	3	140
Keto Bar, Cookies 'n Crème	1 bar (65 g)	24	4	4	240
Keto Bar, Lemon Chiffon	1 bar (65 g)	21	2	4	230
Keto Bar, Mini Lemon Chiffon	1 bar (32 g)	10	1	2	120
Keto Bar, Oatmeal Raisin Crunch	1 bar (56 g)	16	3	1	210
Keto Bar, S'mores	1 bar (65 g)	24	3	5	250
Keto Bar, Strawberry Yogurt	1 bar (65 g)	22	3	4	240

DIET AND NUTRITIONAL BARS, CEREAL BARS

FOOD	SERVING	TOTAL CARBS (G)	NET CARBS (G)	FIBER (G)	CALORIES
Labrada CarbWatchers Lean Body Bar, Chocolate Peanut Butter	1 bar (72 g)	26	1	1	280
Labrada CarbWatchers Lean Body Bar, Texan Pecan Pie	1 bar (72 g)	25	1	t	270
Luna Glow, Chocolate Peanut Crunch	1 bar (35 g)	15	3	1	140
Luna Glow, Fudge Almond Brownie	1 bar (35 g)	15	2	1	140
Luna Glow, Strawberry Caramel Sundae	1 bar (35 g)	15	3	1	140
Met-Rx, Peanut Butter	1 bar (3.5 oz)	50	50	na	344
Myoplex Carb Sense, Apple Cinnamon Delite	1 bar (70 g)	25	4	0	250
Myoplex Carb Sense, Blueberry	1 bar (70 g)	25	2	0	240
Myoplex Carb Sense, Chocolate Dipped Strawberry	1 bar (70 g)	23	1	2	250
Myoplex Carb Sense, Cookies & Cream	1 bar (70 g)	21	2	2	254
Myoplex Carb Sense, Creamy Peanut Butter	1 bar (70 g)	20	2	1	250
Myoplex Carb Sense, Lemon Cheesecake	1 bar (70 g)	22	2	2	240
Nutrilite Positrim Food Bar, Peanut Butter	1 serving (2 bars)	26	26	na	210

DIET AND NUTRITIONAL BARS, CEREAL BARS

FOOD	SERVING	TOTAL CARBS (G)	NET CARBS (G)	FIBER (G)	CALORIES
Odyssey Slim Advantage Protein Bar, Caramel Nut	1 bar (60 g)	23	2	1	240
Odyssey Slim Advantage Protein Bar, Chocolate Coconut Almond	1 bar (60 g)	23	2	2	250
Odyssey Slim Advantage Protein Bar, Rocky Road	1 bar (60 g)	23	2	2	240
PowerBar Pria Carb Select Bar, Caramel Nut	1 bar (48 g)	21	2	2	170
PowerBar Pria Carb Select Bar, Caramel Nut Brownie	1 bar (48 g)	21	2	2	170
PowerBar Pria Carb Select Bar, Cookies n' Caramel	1 bar (48 g)	22	2	2	170
PowerBar Protein Plus Carb Select Bar, Chocolate Peanut Butter	1 bar (70 g)	30	2	2	270
PowerBar Protein Plus Carb Select Bar, Double Chocolate	1 bar (70 g)	30	2	1	260
Promax Carb Conscious Bar, Chocolate Mousse Cake	1 bar (60 g)	21	2	5	240

DIET AND NUTRITIONAL BARS, CEREAL BARS

FOOD	SERVING	TOTAL CARBS (G)	NET CARBS (G)	FIBER (G)	CALORIES
Promax Carb Conscious Bar, Chocolate Peanut Butter	1 bar (60 g)	21	3	5	250
Slim Fast Bar, Chocolate Brownie	1 bar (50 g)	17	2	1	200
Slim Fast Bar, Chocolate Peanut Butter	1 bar (50 g)	17	2	1	200
Slim Fast Bar, Cinnamon Bun	1 bar (50 g)	17	2	0	200
Think Thin! Low Carb Diet Bar, Brownie Crunch	1 bar (60 g)	24	2	2	230
Think Thin! Low Carb Diet Bar, Caramel Swirl	1 bar (60 g)	23	2	0	230
Think Thin! Low Carb Diet Bar, Chocolate Fudge	1 bar (60 g)	22	2	1	240
Think Thin! Low Carb Diet Bar, Chunky Peanut Lite	1 bar (60 g)	22	2	1	250
Think Thin! Low Carb Diet Bar, French Vanilla Latte	1 bar (60 g)	25	2	1	230
Think Thin! Low Carb Diet Bar, French Toast Lite	1 bar (60 g)	22	2	1	240
Think Thin! Low Carb Diet Bar, German Chocolate Coffee Cake	1 bar (60 g)	25	2	1	220

104 DIET AND NUTRITIONAL BARS, CEREAL BARS

FOOD	SERVING	TOTAL CARBS (G)	NET CARBS (G)	FIBER (G)	CALORIES
Think Thin! Low Carb Diet Bar, Lemon Meringue	1 bar (60 g)	20	2	0	230
Think Thin! Low Carb Diet Bar, Mixed Berry	1 bar (60 g)	23	2	0	240
Think Thin! Low Carb Diet Bar, Peanut Butter	1 bar (60 g)	21	2	1	240
Think Thin! Low Carb Diet Bar, S'mores Lite	1 bar (60 g)	23	2	1	240
Ultimate LoCarb 2 Bar, Chocolate Peanut Butter & Jelly	1 bar (60 g)	24	2	0	240
Ultimate LoCarb 2 Bar, Chocolate Smores Supreme	1 bar (60 g)	25	3	0	230
Ultimate LoCarb 2 Bar, Coconut Almond Delight	1 bar (60 g)	26	3	0	250
Ultimate LoCarb 2 Bar, French Vanilla Bean	1 bar (60 g)	24	3	0	240
Viactiv Chocolate Raspberry Crunch	1 bar (1.6 oz)	29	29	na	180
CEREAL AND BREAKFAST BARS					
Atkins Morning Start, Apple Crisp Breakfast Bar	1 bar (37 g)	13	2	6	170

DIET AND NUTRITIONAL BARS, CEREAL BARS

FOOD	SERVING	TOTAL CARBS (G)	NET CARBS (G)	FIBER (G)	CALORIES
Atkins Morning Start, Blueberry Muffin Breakfast Bar	1 bar (40 g)	16	2	7	160
Atkins Morning Start, Chocolate Chip Crisp Breakfast Bar	1 bar (37 g)	14	2	5	140
Atkins Morning Start, Creamy Cinnamon Bun Breakfast Bar	1 bar (40 g)	14	2	6	160
CarboRite Cereal Bar, Blueberry	1 bar (36 g)	22	4	1	110
CarboRite Cereal Bar, Cinnamon Bun	1 bar (36 g)	22	4	1	110
CarboRite Cereal Bar, Strawberry	1 bar (36 g)	22	3	2	110
Carb Well High Protein Cereal Bar, Cinnamon Raisin (Post)	1 bar (35 g)	15	12	3	140
Carb Well High Protein Cereal Bar, Cranberry Almond (Post)	1 bar (35 g)	15	12	3	140
Carb Well High Protein Cereal Bar, Peanut Butter (Post)	1 bar (35 g)	15	12	3	140
Cereal bar, fruit	1 bar (1 oz)	20	19	1	103
Cereal bar, mixed berry	1 bar (1 oz)	20	19.5	.5	104
Chocolate chip crisped rice bar	1 bar (1 oz)	20	19	1	113
Granola bar, hard, almond	1 bar	15	14	1	119
Granola bar, hard, chocolate chip	1 bar	17	16	1	105

DIET AND NUTRITIONAL BARS, CEREAL BARS

FOOD	SERVING	TOTAL CARBS (G)	NET CARBS (G)	FIBER (G)	CALORIES
Granola bar, hard, peanut	1 bar (1 oz)	18	17	1	136
Granola bar, hard, peanut	1 bar (0.85 oz)	15	14	1	116
Granola bar, hard, plain	1 bar (1 oz)	18	17	1	132
Granola bar, soft, chocolate chip w/milk chocolate coating	1 bar (1.25 oz)	22	21	1	163
Granola bar, soft, chocolate chip w/milk chocolate coating	1 bar (1 oz)	18	17	1	130
Granola bar, soft, peanut butter w/milk chocolate coating	1 bar (1.3 oz)	20	19	1	188
Granola bar, soft, chocolate chip, uncoated	1 bar (1.5 oz)	30	28	2	181
Granola bar, soft, chocolate chip, uncoated	1 bar (1 oz)	19	18	1	118
Granola bar, soft, chocolate chip, graham & marshmallow, uncoated	1 bar (1 oz)	20	19	1	120
Granola bar, soft, nut & raisin, uncoated	1 bar (1 oz)	18	16	2	127
Granola bar, soft, peanut butter, uncoated	1 bar (1 oz)	18	17	1	119

FOOD	SERVING	TOTAL CARBS (G)	NET CARBS (G)	FIBER (G)	CALORIES
Granola bar, soft, peanut butter & chocolate chip, uncoated	1 bar (1 oz)	17	16	1	121
Granola bar, soft, plain, uncoated	1 bar (1 oz)	19	18	1	124
Granola bar, soft, raisin, uncoated	1 bar (1.5 oz)	29	27	2	193
Granola bar, soft, raisin, uncoated	1 bar (1 oz)	19	18	1	125

DIPS AND SPREADS

DIPS

FOOD	SERVING	TOTAL CARBS (G)	NET CARBS (G)	FIBER (G)	CALORIES
Atkins French Onion Dip	2 tbsp	1	1	0	30
Atkins Jalapeño Cheddar Dip	2 tbsp	1	1	0	30
Atkins Mild Cheddar Dip	2 tbsp	1	1	0	30
Gringo Billy's Low Carb Guacamole Mix	1 tsp	2	1	1	10
Walden Farms Bacon Dip	2 tbsp	0	0	0	0
Walden Farms French Onion Dip	2 tbsp	0	0	0	0
Walden Farms Ranch Dip	2 tbsp	0	0	0	0

FRUIT SPREADS/TOPPINGS

FOOD	SERVING	TOTAL CARBS (G)	NET CARBS (G)	FIBER (G)	CALORIES
Keto Fruit Spread, Apricot	1 tbsp	4	3	1	15
Keto Fruit Spread, Blackberry & Apple	1 tbsp	2	3	1	17

DIPS AND SPREADS

FOOD	SERVING	TOTAL CARBS (G)	NET CARBS (G)	FIBER (G)	CALORIES
Keto Fruit Spread, Black Currant	1 tbsp	2	3	1	10
Keto Fruit Spread, Blueberry	1 tbsp	4	3	1	15
Keto Fruit Spread, Grape	1 tbsp	4	3	1	15
Keto Fruit Spread, Orange Marmalade	1 tbsp	4	3	1	15
Keto Fruit Spread, Pineapple	1 tbsp	2	3	1	17
Keto Fruit Spread, Raspberry	1 tbsp	4	3	1	15
Keto Fruit Spread, Strawberry	1 tbsp	4	3	1	15
La Nouba Fruit Spread, Apricot	1 tbsp	10	1.6	0	40.8
La Nouba Fruit Spread, Blueberry	1 tbsp	10	1.6	0	40.8
La Nouba Fruit Spread, Orange Marmalade	1 tbsp	10	1.6	0	40.8
La Nouba Fruit Spread, Raspberry	1 tbsp	10	1.6	0	40.8
La Nouba Fruit Spread, Strawberry	1 tbsp	10	1.6	0	40.8
La Nouba Hazelnut Chocolate Spread	1 tbsp	4.8	0	na	108
Steel's Marion Blackberry Fruit Spread	1 tbsp	2	2	0	10

FOOD	SERVING	TOTAL CARBS (G)	NET CARBS (G)	FIBER (G)	CALORIES
Steel's Strawberry Fruit Spread	1 tbsp	1.5	1.5	0	6
Sugar Free TWIST Chocolate Spread	2 tbsp	20	0	2	167
Sugar Free TWIST Hazelnut Chocolate Spread	2 tbsp	20	1.6	1.4	117
EGGS					
Egg, fried	1 large	1	1	0	92
Egg, omelet	1 large	1	1	0	93
Egg, scrambled	1 large	1	1	0	101
Egg substitute, liquid	¼ cup	t	t	0	53
Egg white	2 large	t	t	0	33
Egg white, dried powder	1 tbsp	1	1	0	53
Egg, whole, fresh	1 extra large	1	1	0	86
Egg, whole, fresh	1 jumbo	1	1	0	97
Egg, whole, fresh	1 large	1	1	0	75
Egg, whole, fresh	1 medium	.5	.5	0	66
Egg, whole, fresh	1 small	t	t	0	55
Egg, whole, hard boiled	1 large	t	t	0	78
Egg, whole, poached	1 large	t	t	0	75

ENTRÉES, DINNERS AND SIDES, BY BRAND
FROZEN AND READY MEALS
ATKINS, ENTRÉES

FOOD	SERVING	TOTAL CARBS (G)	NET CARBS (G)	FIBER (G)	CALORIES
Beef Stroganoff	½ tray (5 oz)	9	5	4	210
Chicken Marsala	½ tray (5 oz)	10	6	4	180

ENTRÉES

FOOD	SERVING	TOTAL CARBS (G)	NET CARBS (G)	FIBER (G)	CALORIES
Four Cheese Macaroni & Cheese	½ tray (5 oz)	9	7	3	250
Meat Loaf	½ tray (5 oz)	2	2	0	290
Heat-and-Serve Entrée, Bacon & Onion Crustless Quiche	1 quiche	2	2	0	320
Heat-and-Serve Entrée, Four Cheese Crustless Quiche	1 quiche	2	2	0	290
Heat-and-Serve Entrée, Smoked Ham & Cheese Crustless Quiche	1 quiche	2	2	0	290
Italian Frozen Entrée, Baked Ziti	½ tray (5 oz)	10	6	4	200
Soufflé, Cheddar & Bacon	1 souffle	3	3	1	200
Soufflé, Crab & Cheddar	1 souffle	4	2	2	290
Soufflé, Spinach, Tomato & Feta	1 souffle	4	2	2	170
CARB'TASTIC					
Penne Alfredo	1 package	25	4	21	280
Penne w/"Meat" Sauce	1 package	22	8	14	240
Vegetarian Chili Mac	1 package	19	5	14	290
Vegetarian Pesto Primavera	1 package	22	8	14	270
Vegetarian Teriyaki	1 package	29	9	20	220

ENTRÉES

FOOD	SERVING	TOTAL CARBS (G)	NET CARBS (G)	FIBER (G)	CALORIES
STOUFFER'S LEAN CUISINE, CAFÉ CLASSICS					
Baked Chicken	1 serving	32	30	2	230
Baked Fish	1 serving	40	38	2	290
Beef Peppercorn	1 serving	25	22	3	220
Beef Portabello	1 serving	25	22	3	220
Beef Pot Roast	1 serving	25	23	2	200
Bow Tie Pasta & Chicken	1 serving	31	28	3	220
Cheese Lasagna w/Chicken	1 serving	36	33	3	280
Chicken à l'Orange	1 serving	35	33	2	230
Chicken & Vegetables	1 serving	33	30	3	250
Chicken Carbonara	1 serving	31	29	2	270
Chicken in Peanut Sauce	1 serving	32	30	2	280
Chicken Marsala	1 serving	12	9	3	140
Chicken Mediterranean	1 serving	38	34	4	260
Chicken Parmesan	1 serving	36	34	2	270
Chicken Piccata	1 serving	41	40	1	270
Chicken w/Basil Cream Sauce	1 serving	30	28	2	260
Chicken w/Almonds	1 serving	38	36	2	260
Fiesta Grilled Chicken	1 serving	31	28	3	260
Glazed Chicken	1 serving	25	24	1	230
Glazed Turkey Tenderloins	1 serving	39	35	4	270
Grilled Chicken	1 serving	15	11	4	160
Herb Roasted Chicken	1 serving	23	20	3	190
Honey Mustard Chicken	1 serving	37	36	1	260
Honey Roasted Pork	1 serving	34	31	3	230
Meatloaf & Whipped Potatoes	1 serving	30	27	3	270

ENTRÉES

FOOD	SERVING	TOTAL CARBS (G)	NET CARBS (G)	FIBER (G)	CALORIES
Orange Beef	1 serving	42	40	2	300
Oriental Beef	1 serving	33	31	2	210
Oven Roasted Beef	1 serving	18	16	2	210
Roasted Garlic Chicken	1 serving	28	27	1	230
Roasted Turkey Breast	1 serving	51	48	3	270
Salisbury Steak	1 serving	24	21	3	270
Sesame Chicken	1 serving	48	46	2	320
Shrimp & Angel Hair Pasta	1 serving	34	32	2	240
Southern Beef Tips	1 serving	37	34	3	250
Sweet+Sour Chicken	1 serving	51	50	1	290
Teriyaki Chicken	1 serving	42	42	0	280
Deluxe Pizza	1 serving	55	52	3	370
Four Cheese Pizza	1 serving	60	57	3	380
Pepperoni Pizza	1 serving	55	52	3	380
Roasted Vegetable Pizza	1 serving	57	54	3	330
Thai-Style Chicken	1 serving	35	34	1	250

STOUFFER'S LEAN CUISINE, EVERYDAY FAVORITES

FOOD	SERVING	TOTAL CARBS (G)	NET CARBS (G)	FIBER (G)	CALORIES
Alfredo Pasta w/ Chicken & Broccoli	1 serving	38	35	3	270
Angel Hair Pasta	1 serving	48	44	4	260
Baked Chicken Florentine	1 serving	25	23	2	190
Cheese Cannelloni	1 serving	31	28	3	240
Cheese Lasagna Florentine Bake	1 serving	37	34	3	270
Cheese Ravioli	1 serving	38	35	3	250
Chicken Chow Mein	1 serving	35	33	2	230
Chicken Enchilada	1 serving	48	45	3	290

ENTRÉES 113

FOOD	SERVING	TOTAL CARBS (G)	NET CARBS (G)	FIBER (G)	CALORIES
Chicken Fettucini	1 serving	34	32	2	270
Chicken Florentine Lasagna	1 serving	36	33	3	270
Five Cheese Lasagna	1 serving	44	40	4	310
Cheddar Potato	1 serving	35	30	5	260
Fettucini Alfredo	1 serving	40	38	2	280
Honey Dijon Grilled Chicken	1 serving	25	22	3	230
Hunan Beef & Broccoli	1 serving	36	35	1	230
Lasagna w/Meat Sauce	1 serving	43	40	3	310
Macaroni & Beef	1 serving	38	35	3	270
Macaroni & Cheese	1 serving	42	41	1	300
Mandarin Chicken	1 serving	46	44	2	270
Oriental Style Pot Stickers	1 serving	55	52	3	320
Penne Pasta w/Tomato	1 serving	50	50	5	270
Roasted Chicken	1 serving	33	31	2	260
Roasted Potatoes w/Broccoli	1 serving	37	33	4	240
Roasted Turkey & Vegetables	1 serving	13	9	4	120
Santa Fe Rice & Beans	1 serving	53	48	5	300
Spaghetti w/Meat Sauce	1 serving	35	32	3	240
Spaghetti w/Meatballs	1 serving	37	34	3	260
Steak Tips Portabello	1 serving	13	10	3	130
Stuffed Cabbage	1 serving	26	22	4	190
Swedish Meatballs	1 serving	36	34	2	290
Teriyaki Stir-Fry	1 serving	49	46	3	300
Three Bean Chili	1 serving	43	35	8	270

ENTRÉES

FOOD	SERVING	TOTAL CARBS (G)	NET CARBS (G)	FIBER (G)	CALORIES
Three Cheese Chicken	1 serving	15	13	2	190
Vegetable Eggroll	1 serving	62	59	3	330

STOUFFER'S LEAN CUISINE, DINNERTIME SELECTIONS

FOOD	SERVING	TOTAL CARBS (G)	NET CARBS (G)	FIBER (G)	CALORIES
Beef Steak Tips Dijon	1 serving	44	39	5	310
Chicken Fettucini	1 serving	51	46	5	380
Chicken Florentine	1 serving	53	47	6	370
Glazed Chicken	1 serving	39	36	3	310
Grilled Chicken & Penne Pasta	1 serving	46	41	5	340
Grilled Chicken Tuscan	1 serving	34	31	3	270
Jumbo Rigatoni	1 serving	50	44	6	390
Oriental Glazed Chicken	1 serving	58	56	2	330
Roasted Chicken	1 serving	48	44	4	320
Roasted Turkey Breast	1 serving	50	46	6	340
Salisbury Steak	1 serving	35	29	6	320

STOUFFER'S LEAN CUISINE, SKILLET SENSATIONS

FOOD	SERVING	TOTAL CARBS (G)	NET CARBS (G)	FIBER (G)	CALORIES
Beef Teriyaki & Rice	1 serving	31	29	2	180
Chicken Alfredo	1 serving	23	21	2	180
Chicken Oriental	1 serving	23	21	2	170
Chicken Primavera	1 serving	28	27	1	180
Chicken Teriyaki	1 serving	37	33	4	230
Garlic Chicken	1 serving	36	34	2	240
Herb Chicken & Roasted Potatoes	1 serving	24	22	2	170
Roasted Turkey	1 serving	23	20	3	130
Three Cheese Chicken	1 serving	26	24	2	200

STOUFFER'S LEAN CUISINE, CAFÉ CLASSICS BOWLS

FOOD	SERVING	TOTAL CARBS (G)	NET CARBS (G)	FIBER (G)	CALORIES
Chicken Fried Rice Bowl	1 serving	64	60	4	410
Chicken Teriyaki Bowl	1 serving	63	61	2	340

ENTRÉES

FOOD	SERVING	TOTAL CARBS (G)	NET CARBS (G)	FIBER (G)	CALORIES
Creamy Chicken & Vegetables Bowl	1 serving	45	42	3	310
Grilled Chicken Caesar Bowl	1 serving	30	36	4	240
Teriyaki Steak Bowl	1 serving	48	44	4	340
Three Cheese Stuffed Rigatoni Bowl	1 serving	46	42	4	280
INSTANT MIXES					
ATKINS SAVORY SIDES					
Pilaf Style Broccoli Au Gratin	½ cup	9	4	5	79
Pilaf Style Cheese & Chives	½ cup	9	4	5	61
Pilaf Style Creamy Mushroom	½ cup	9	4	5	75
Pilaf Style Mexican Fiesta	½ cup	9	4	5	57
Pilaf Style Stir Fry	½ cup	9	4	5	61
CARB OPTIONS					
Classic Basil Pesto Pasta Side Dish	¾ cup	12	8	4	220
Sundried Tomato Pesto Pasta Side Dish	¾ cup	12	8	4	160
KETO					
Ketato, Bacon, Cheddar & Chives Flavor, Dehydrated Potato Mix	¼ pkt	11	5	6	90

ENTRÉES

FOOD	SERVING	TOTAL CARBS (G)	NET CARBS (G)	FIBER (G)	CALORIES
Ketato, Classic Flavor, Dehydrated Potato Mix	¼ pkt	11	5	6	90
Ketato, Garlic Parmesan Flavor, Dehydrated Potato Mix	¼ pkt	11	5	6	90
Ketato, Sour Cream & Cheddar Flavor, Dehydrated Potato Mix	¼ pkt	11	5	6	90
Ketato, Sweet Potato Flavor, Dehydrated Potato Mix	¼ pkt	11	5	6	90

ENTRÉES, DINNERS AND SIDES, GENERIC

CANNED

FOOD	SERVING	TOTAL CARBS (G)	NET CARBS (G)	FIBER (G)	CALORIES
Beef ravioli in tomato & meat sauce	1 serving	37	33	4	229
Beef ravioli in tomato & meat sauce, mini ravioli	1 serving	41	39	3	239
Beef stew	1 serving	16	12	4	218
Chicken & dumplings, canned	1 serving	23	20	3	218
Chow mein, no noodles or rice	2 cups	12	6	6	160
Corned beef hash	1 cup	22	19	3	387
Macaroni w/beef in tomato sauce	1 serving	31	28	3	184
Macaroni & cheese	1 serving	29	26	3	199

ENTRÉES

FOOD	SERVING	TOTAL CARBS (G)	NET CARBS (G)	FIBER (G)	CALORIES
Roast beef hash	1 cup	23	19	4	385
Spaghetti & meatballs in tomato sauce	1 serving	34	32	2	250
Sweet & sour vegetables, fruit & sauce w/chicken	1 serving	32	32	na	165
FROZEN					
Beef macaroni	1 serving	33	28	5	211
Beef pot pie	1 serving	44	42	2	449
Beef strips w/Oriental-style vegetables	1 serving	71	71	na	433
Beef Stroganoff & noodles w/carrots & peas	1 serving	59	55	4	600
Chicken Alfredo w/fettucini & vegetables	1 serving	33	29	4	373
Chicken cordon bleu, filled w/cheese & ham	1 serving	15	15	na	344
Chicken enchilada & Mexican-style rice w/Monterey Jack cheese sauce	1 serving	48	43	5	376
Chicken fajita	1 serving	17	17	na	129
Chicken mesquite w/barbeque, corn medley, potatoes au gratin	1 serving	45	41	4	321
Chicken pot pie	1 serving	43	41	2	484

ENTRÉES

FOOD	SERVING	TOTAL CARBS (G)	NET CARBS (G)	FIBER (G)	CALORIES
Creamed chipped beef	1 serving	7	7	na	175
Dinner-type meal (TV), generic, frozen	1 meal (16 oz)	54	48	6	512
Fried chicken w/mashed potatoes & corn in sauce	1 serving	35	33	2	470
Entrée or meal (8–11 oz), less than 340 calories	1 carton (9.5 oz)	40	37	3	298
Escalloped chicken & noodles	1 serving	31	31	na	419
Fried chicken meal w/mashed potatoes, corn in seasoned sauce	1 serving	35	33	2	470
Italian sausage lasagna	1 serving	40	37	3	456
Lasagna w/meat & sauce	1 serving	26	23	3	277
Meat loaf dinner w/tomato sauce, mashed potatoes & carrots in seasoned sauce	1 serving	34	28	6	612
Mesquite beef w/barbeque sauce, mashed potatoes, & sweetened corn	1 serving	38	33	5	320
Mexican style dinner w/tamales, beef enchiladas & chili sauce, beans & rice	1 serving	68	60	8	508

ENTRÉES

FOOD	SERVING	TOTAL CARBS (G)	NET CARBS (G)	FIBER (G)	CALORIES
Roasted chicken w/garlic sauce, pasta & vegetable medley	1 serving	22	18	4	214
Salisbury steak in gravy, w/macaroni & cheese	1 serving	26	26	na	386
Salisbury steak in gravy, w/mashed potatoes & corn in seasoned sauce	1 serving	47	40	7	782
Sliced beef meal, w/gravy, mashed potatoes & peas in seasoned sauce	1 serving	19	15	4	270
Stuffed peppers w/beef, in tomato sauce	1 serving	21	16	5	189
Tuna noodle casserole	1 cup	34	32	2	259
Turkey & gravy w/dressing & broccoli	1 serving	52	52	0	504
Turkey & gravy w/dressing meal, w/mashed potatoes & corn in seasoned sauce	1 serving	34	31	3	280
Turkey pot pie	1 serving	70	66	4	699
Veal parmigiana meal w/tomato sauce, mashed potatoes & peas in seasoned sauce	1 serving	35	28	7	362

FAST FOOD AND OTHER RESTAURANTS

APPETIZERS

DENNY'S

FOOD	SERVING	TOTAL CARBS (G)	NET CARBS (G)	FIBER (G)	CALORIES
Sampler	1 serving	124	120	4	1,405
Buffalo Wings	9 wings	11	9	2	974
Mozzarella Sticks	8 sticks	49	43	6	710
Smothered Cheese Fries	1 serving	69	69	0	767
Buffalo Chicken Strips	5 strips	43	43	0	734
Chicken Strips	5 strips	56	56	0	720
Nacho	1 serving	117	106	11	1,278
Mini-Burgers w/Onion Rings	8 burgers	179	169	10	2,044

RUBY TUESDAY

FOOD	SERVING	TOTAL CARBS (G)	NET CARBS (G)	FIBER (G)	CALORIES
Super Sampler	1 serving	na	16	3	275
Tuesday's Sampler	1 serving	na	13	1	199
Three Cheese Spinach Dip & Chips	1 serving	na	20	2	288
Veggies & Dip, Low Carb	1 serving	na	3	2	28
Loaded Cheese Fries	1 serving	na	17	4	282
Chicken Quesadilla	1 serving	na	12	1	225
Chicken Quesadilla Low Carb	1 serving	na	3	2	183
Queso & Chips	1 serving	na	21	2	318
Spicy Buffalo Wings, Low Carb	1 serving	na	1	0	228
Boneless Buffalo Wings	1 serving	na	7	0	166
Spicy Honey BBQ Tenders	1 serving	na	13	0	138

FAST FOOD AND OTHER RESTAURANTS

FOOD	SERVING	TOTAL CARBS (G)	NET CARBS (G)	FIBER (G)	CALORIES
Chicken Tenders	1 serving	na	6	0	108
Fried Cheese Sticks	1 serving	na	11	2	172
BEVERAGES AND SHAKES					
ARBY'S					
Milk	8 oz	12	12	0	120
Hot Chocolate	8.6 oz	23	23	0	110
Orange Juice	10 oz	34	34	0	140
Vanilla Shake	14 oz	83	83	0	470
Chocolate Shake	14 oz	84	84	0	480
Strawberry Shake	14 oz	87	87	0	500
Jamocha	14 oz	82	82	0	470
BURGER KING					
Vanilla Milk Shake	1 small (298 g)	57	57	0	400
Vanilla Milk Shake	1 medium (397 g)	76	76	0	540
Vanilla Milk Shake	1 large (588 g)	113	113	t	800
Chocolate Milk Shake, Syrup Added	1 small (284 g)	65	65	t	410
Chocolate Milk Shake, Syrup Added	1 medium (397 g)	97	95	2	600
Chocolate Milk Shake, Syrup Added	1 large (581 g)	133	131	2	850
Strawberry Milk Shake, Syrup Added	1 small (284 g)	64	64	0	410
Strawberry Milk Shake, Syrup Added	1 medium (397 g)	96	96	0	590
Strawberry Milk Shake, Syrup Added	1 large (581 g)	131	131	t	840
DAIRY QUEEN					
Chocolate Malt, Small	1 small	111	110	1	640

FAST FOOD AND OTHER RESTAURANTS

FOOD	SERVING	TOTAL CARBS (G)	NET CARBS (G)	FIBER (G)	CALORIES
Chocolate Malt, Medium	1 medium	153	151	2	870
Chocolate Malt, Large	1 large	222	220	2	1,320
Chocolate Shake, Small	1 small	93	92	1	560
Chocolate Shake, Medium	1 medium	129	127	2	760
Chocolate Shake, Large	1 large	186	184	2	1,140
Misty Slush, Small	1 small	56	56	0	220
Misty Slush, Medium	1 medium	74	74	0	290
DENNY'S					
MilkShake, Vanilla or Chocolate	12 oz cup	76	76	t	560
Malted MilkShake, Vanilla or Chocolate	12 oz cup	82	82	t	583
Floats, Root Beer or Cola	12 oz cup	47	47	0	280
Oreo Blender Blaster	15 oz cup	112	110	2	895
Oreo Blender Blaster for Kids	10 oz cup	72	71	1	580
HARDEE'S					
Vanilla Shake, Regular	16 fl oz	99	89	10	580
Vanilla Shake, Large	20 fl oz	123	111	12	730
Chocolate Shake, Regular	16 fl oz	137	125	12	710
Chocolate Shake, Large	20 fl oz	171	157	14	880
Strawberry Shake, Regular	16 fl oz	139	129	10	720

FOOD	SERVING	TOTAL CARBS (G)	NET CARBS (G)	FIBER (G)	CALORIES
Strawberry Shake, Large	20 fl oz	174	163	11	890
JACK IN THE BOX					
Creamy Caramel Ice Cream Shake, Small	1 shake	87	87	0	670
Creamy Caramel Ice Cream Shake, Medium	1 shake	109	109	0	860
Creamy Caramel Ice Cream Shake, Large	1 shake	173	172	1	1,330
Chocolate Ice Cream Shake, Small	1 shake	89	88	1	660
Chocolate Ice Cream Shake, Medium	1 shake	111	110	1	850
Chocolate Ice Cream Shake, Large	1 shake	178	176	2	1,310
Oreo Cookie Ice Cream Shake, Small	1 shake	81	80	1	670
Oreo Cookie Ice Cream Shake, Medium	1 shake	103	102	1	870
Oreo Cookie Ice Cream Shake, Large	1 shake	161	159	2	1,350
Strawberry Ice Cream Shake, Small	1 shake	84	84	0	640
Strawberry Ice Cream Shake, Medium	1 shake	106	106	0	830
Strawberry Ice Cream Shake, Large	1 shake	167	167	0	1,270
Strawberry Banana Ice Cream Shake, Small	1 shake	100	100	0	700
Strawberry Banana Ice Cream Shake, Medium	1 shake	122	122	0	900

FAST FOOD AND OTHER RESTAURANTS

FOOD	SERVING	TOTAL CARBS (G)	NET CARBS (G)	FIBER (G)	CALORIES
Strawberry Banana Ice Cream Shake, Large	1 shake	199	199	0	1,410
Vanilla Ice Cream Shake, Small	1 shake	65	65	0	570
Vanilla Ice Cream Shake, Medium	1 shake	85	85	0	750
Vanilla Ice Cream Shake, Large	1 shake	129	129	0	1,140
MCDONALD'S					
Chocolate Triple Thick Shake	12 fl oz	70	69	1	430
Chocolate Triple Thick Shake	16 fl oz	94	93	1	580
Chocolate Triple Thick Shake	21 fl oz	123	121	2	750
Chocolate Triple Thick Shake	32 fl oz	187	184	3	1,150
Strawberry Triple Thick Shake	12 fl oz	67	67	t	420
Strawberry Triple Thick Shake	16 fl oz	89	89	t	560
Strawberry Triple Thick Shake	21 fl oz	116	115	1	730
Strawberry Triple Thick Shake	32 fl oz	178	176	2	1,120
Vanilla Triple Thick Shake	12 fl oz	67	67	0	430
Vanilla Triple Thick Shake	16 fl oz	89	89	0	570
Vanilla Triple Thick Shake	21 fl oz	116	116	0	750

FOOD	SERVING	TOTAL CARBS (G)	NET CARBS (G)	FIBER (G)	CALORIES
Vanilla Triple Thick Shake	32 fl oz	178	178	t	1,140
SONIC					
Coconut Cream Pie Shake, Regular	1 shake	79	78	1	721
Coconut Cream Pie Shake, Large	1 shake	116	115	1	1,004
Chocolate Cream Pie Shake, Regular	1 shake	96	95	1	795
Chocolate Cream Pie Shake, Large	1 shake	151	150	1	1,151
Banana Cream Pie Shake, Regular	1 shake	92	90	2	775
Banana Cream Pie Shake, Large	1 shake	130	128	3	1,058
Chocolate Shake, Regular	1 shake	58	58	0	564
Chocolate Shake, Large	1 shake	77	77	0	752
Strawberry Shake, Regular	1 shake	46	45	1	510
Strawberry Shake, Large	1 shake	61	60	1	680
Vanilla Shake, Regular	1 shake	32	32	0	454
Vanilla Shake, Large	1 shake	42	42	0	605
Banana Shake, Regular	1 shake	46	45	1	508
Banana Shake, Large	1 shake	70	67	3	713
Pineapple Shake, Regular	1 shake	74	73	1	615
Pineapple Shake, Large	1 shake	99	98	1	820

FAST FOOD AND OTHER RESTAURANTS

FOOD	SERVING	TOTAL CARBS (G)	NET CARBS (G)	FIBER (G)	CALORIES
Reese's Sonic Blast Shake, Regular	1 shake	52	51	1	658
Reese's Sonic Blast Shake, Large	1 shake	78	76	2	963
M&M Sonic Blast Shake, Regular	1 shake	58	57	1	641
M&M Sonic Blast Shake, Large	1 shake	89	87	2	931
Oreo Sonic Blast Shake, Regular	1 shake	57	56	1	638
Oreo Sonic Blast Shake, Large	1 shake	88	86	2	927
Butterfinger Sonic Blast Shake, Regular	1 shake	56	55	1	636
Butterfinger Sonic Blast Shake, Large	1 shake	85	83	2	924
Add 1 oz Malt to Any Shake	1 oz	22	22	0	104
WENDY'S					
Frosty, Junior	6 oz	28	28	0	160
Frosty, Small	12 oz	56	56	0	160
Frosty, Medium	16 oz	74	74	0	430
BREAKFAST ITEMS					
ARBY'S					
Biscuit w/Butter	1 biscuit (2.9 oz)	27	26.5	.5	280
Biscuit w/Ham	1 biscuit (4.3 oz)	28	27	1	330
Biscuit w/Sausage	1 biscuit (4.2 oz)	27	26	1	440
Biscuit w/Bacon	1 biscuit (3.2 oz)	27	26	1	320
Croissant w/Ham	1 croissant (3.7 oz)	29	29	0	310
Croissant w/Sausage	1 croissant (3.6 oz)	28	28	0	420

FAST FOOD AND OTHER RESTAURANTS

FOOD	SERVING	TOTAL CARBS (G)	NET CARBS (G)	FIBER (G)	CALORIES
Croissant w/Bacon	1 croissant (2.5 oz)	28	28	0	300
Sourdough w/Ham	1 biscuit (4 oz)	30	29	1	220
Sourdough w/Sausage	1 biscuit (4 oz)	29	28	1	330
Sourdough w/Bacon	1 biscuit (5 oz)	29	27	2	3,809
Add Egg	1 egg (2 oz)	2	2	0	110
Add Slice Swiss Cheese	1 slice (.5 oz)	3	3	0	45
French Toastix	1 serving (4.4 oz)	48	44	4	370
BURGER KING					
Croissan'wich w/Bacon, Egg & Cheese	1 croissant (119 g)	25	25	t	360
Croissan'wich w/Ham, Egg & Cheese	1 croissant (146 g)	25	25	t	360
Croissan'wich w/ Sausage, Egg & Cheese	1 croissant (157 g)	24	23	1	520
Croissan'wich w/ Sausage & Cheese	1 croissant (107 g)	23	23	t	420
Croissan'wich w/ Egg & Cheese	1 croissant (112 g)	24	24	t	320
French Toast Sticks	5 sticks	46	44	2	390
Hash Brown Rounds	1 small size	23	21	2	230
Hash Brown Rounds	1 large size	38	34	4	390
CHICK-FIL-A					
Plain Biscuit	1 biscuit (2.75 g)	38	37	1	260
Hot Buttered Biscuit	1 biscuit (2.78 g)	38	37	1	270
Chick-fil-A Chicken Biscuit	1 biscuit (4.83 g)	43	41	2	400
Chick-fil-A Chicken Biscuit w/Cheese	1 biscuit (5.32 g)	43	41	2	450
Biscuit w/Bacon	1 biscuit (3.02 g)	38	37	1	300

FAST FOOD AND OTHER RESTAURANTS

FOOD	SERVING	TOTAL CARBS (G)	NET CARBS (G)	FIBER (G)	CALORIES
Biscuit w/Bacon & Egg	1 biscuit (5.02 g)	38	37	1	390
Biscuit w/Bacon, Egg & Cheese	1 biscuit (5.48 g)	38	37	1	430
Biscuit w/Egg	1 biscuit (4.75 g)	38	37	1	340
Biscuit w/Egg & Cheese	1 biscuit (5.21 g)	38	37	1	390
Biscuit w/Sausage	1 biscuit (4.2 g)	42	41	1	410
Biscuit w/Sausage & Egg	1 biscuit (6.2 g)	43	42	1	500
Biscuit w/Sausage, Egg & Cheese	1 biscuit (6.6 g)	43	42	1	540
Biscuit w/Gravy	1 biscuit (6.75 g)	44	43	1	310
Hash Browns	1 serving (2.98 g)	20	18	2	170
Danish	1 bun (4.6 g)	63	61	2	430
DENNY'S					
Slim Slam w/o Topping, Fit Fare Item	1 serving	39	38	1	421
Carb-Watch Two Egg & Three Meat Breakfast	1 serving	10	9	1	653
Ultimate Carb-Watch Omelette	1 serving	11	9	2	662
Carb-Watch Ham & Cheddar Omelette	1 serving	8	7	1	610
One Egg	1 serving	t	1	0	120
Two Egg Breakfast w/Hash Browns	1 serving	24	22	2	825
Egg Beaters Egg Substitute	1 serving	2	2	0	56

FAST FOOD AND OTHER RESTAURANTS

FOOD	SERVING	TOTAL CARBS (G)	NET CARBS (G)	FIBER (G)	CALORIES
Ham, Grilled, Sliced, Honey Smoked	1 serving	6	6	0	85
Bacon	4 strips	1	1	0	162
Sausage	4 links	0	0	0	354
Toast, Dry	1 slice	17	16	1	90
English Muffin, Dry	1 muffin	24	23	1	125
Bagel, Dry	1 bagel	46	46	0	235
Biscuit	1 biscuit	22	22	0	192
Quaker Oatmeal	4 oz serving	18	15	3	100
Kellogg's Dry Cereal	1 oz serving	23	22	1	100
Musselman's Apple Sauce	1 serving	15	14	1	60
Banana	1 banana	29	25	4	110
Honeydew Mellon	¼ mellon	8	7	1	31
Canteloupe	¼ mellon	8	7	1	32
Grapefruit	½ grapefruit	16	10	6	60
Grapes	3 oz	15	14	1	55
Meat Lover's Skillet	1 serving	27	17	10	1,031
Meat Lover's Breakfast	1 serving	72	69	3	1,027
Chicken Fajita Skillet	1 serving	30	19	11	855
Original Grand Slam	1 serving	33	31	2	665
All American Slam	1 serving	3	2	1	816
French Slam	1 serving	71	69	3	1,119
Farmer's Slam	1 serving	82	79	3	1,200
Grand Slam Slugger	1 serving	74	71	3	927
Lumberjack Slam w/Hash Browns	1 serving	73	70	3	1,035
Corned Beef Hash Slam	1 serving	11	10	1	668
Ultimate Omelette	1 serving	8	7	1	619

FAST FOOD AND OTHER RESTAURANTS

FOOD	SERVING	TOTAL CARBS (G)	NET CARBS (G)	FIBER (G)	CALORIES
Veggie-Cheese Omelette	1 serving	11	9	2	494
Veggie-Cheese Omelette w/Eggbeaters	1 serving	11	8	3	346
Ham & Cheddar Omelette	1 serving	5	5	0	595
Ham & Cheddar Omelette w/Eggbeaters	1 serving	5	5	0	468
Oatmeal Deluxe	19 oz serving	95	88	7	460
Oatmeal	4 oz serving	18	15	3	100
Country Fried Steak & Eggs	1 serving	13	7	6	464
T-Bone Steak & Eggs	1 serving	1	0	1	991
Sirloin Steak & Eggs	1 serving	1	0	1	675
Breakfast Dagwood	1 serving	81	80	1	1,446
Moons Over My Hammy	1 serving	42	40	2	841
Belgian Waffle Platter w/o Meat	1 serving	28	28	0	619
Fabulous French Toast Platter w/o Meat	1 serving	104	101	3	1,146
Buttermilk Pancake Platter w/o Meat	1 serving	47	45	2	466
Buttermilk Pancake w/o Meat	1 serving	47	45	2	223
Country Fried Potatoes	1 serving	23	13	10	394
Hash Browns	1 serving	20	18	2	197
Hash Browns, Covered	1 serving	21	19	2	280
Hash Browns, Covered & Smothered	1 serving	54	51	3	493
Fresh Fruit Bowl w/Bagel	1 serving	86	81	5	407
Grits	4 oz serving	18	18	0	80

FAST FOOD AND OTHER RESTAURANTS

FOOD	SERVING	TOTAL CARBS (G)	NET CARBS (G)	FIBER (G)	CALORIES
HARDEE'S					
Breakfast Bowl, Low Carb	1 serving	6	4	2	620
Made from Scratch Biscuit	1 biscuit	35	35	0	370
Bacon Biscuit	1 biscuit	37	37	0	560
Sausage Biscuit	1 biscuit	36	36	0	530
Country Ham Biscuit	1 biscuit	36	36	0	440
Chicken Fillet Biscuit	1 biscuit	50	49	1	600
Country Steak Biscuit	1 biscuit	44	44	0	620
Smoked Sausage Biscuit	1 biscuit	37	37	0	620
Sausage & Egg Biscuit	1 biscuit	36	36	0	610
Bacon, Egg & Cheese Biscuit	1 biscuit	37	37	0	560
Ham, Egg & Cheese Biscuit	1 biscuit	37	37	0	560
Loaded Omelet Biscuit	1 biscuit	36	36	0	500
Biscuit N Gravy	1 biscuit	47	47	0	530
Sunrise Croissant w/Ham	1 biscuit	28	28	0	430
Sunrise Croissant w/Bacon	1 biscuit	28	28	0	450
Sunrise Croissant w/Sausage Patty	1 biscuit	29	29	0	550
Frisco Breakfast Sandwich	1 sandwich	38	36	2	360
Tortilla Scrambler	1 serving	18	18	0	310
Big Country Breakfast Platter, Country Ham	1 platter	90	87	3	970

FAST FOOD AND OTHER RESTAURANTS

FOOD	SERVING	TOTAL CARBS (G)	NET CARBS (G)	FIBER (G)	CALORIES
Big Country Breakfast Platter, Breakfast Ham	1 platter	90	87	3	970
Big Country Breakfast Platter, Bacon	1 platter	90	87	3	980
Big Country Breakfast Platter, Sausage	1 platter	91	87	4	1,060
Big Country Breakfast Platter, Chicken	1 platter	105	101	4	1,140
Big Country Breakfast Platter, Country Steak	1 platter	98	94	4	1,150
Pancakes	3 pancakes	55	53	2	300
JACK IN THE BOX					
Breakfast Jack	1 serving	34	34	0	305
Extreme Sausage Sandwich	1 serving	37	37	0	690
French Toast Sticks	1 serving	89	87	2	560
Hash Browns	1 serving	13	11	2	150
Sausage Biscuit	1 serving	41	39	2	600
Sausage Croissant	1 serving	42	41	1	605
Sausage, Egg & Cheese Biscuit	1 serving	50	48	2	970
Sourdough Breakfast Sandwich	1 serving	37	35	2	445
Supreme Croissant	1 serving	41	40	1	475
Ultimate Breakfast Sandwich	1 serving	58	56	2	605
MCDONALD'S					
Egg McMuffin	1 serving	28	26	2	300
Sausage McMuffin	1 serving	28	26	2	370

FOOD	SERVING	TOTAL CARBS (G)	NET CARBS (G)	FIBER (G)	CALORIES
Sausage McMuffin w/Egg	1 serving	29	27	2	450
English Muffin	1 muffin	27	25	2	150
Bacon, Egg & Cheese Biscuit	1 serving	32	31	1	460
Sausage Biscuit w/Egg	1 serving	31	30	1	490
Sausage Biscuit	1 serving	30	29	1	410
Biscuit	1 biscuit	30	29	1	240
Bacon, Egg & Cheese McGriddles	1 serving	43	42	1	440
Sausage, Egg & Cheese McGriddles	1 serving	43	42	1	550
Sausage McGriddles	1 serving	42	41	1	420
Ham, Egg & Cheese Bagel	1 serving	58	56	2	550
Spanish Omelette Bagel	1 serving	59	56	3	710
Steak, Egg & Cheese Bagel	1 serving	57	55	2	640
Bagel, Plain	1 bagel	54	52	2	260
Big Breakfast	1 serving	45	42	3	700
Deluxe Breakfast	1 serving	130	127	3	1,190
Sausage Burrito	1 burrito	24	22	2	290
Hotcakes & Sausage	1 serving	104	104	0	780
Hotcakes w/Margarine & Syrup	1 serving	104	104	0	600
Sausage	1 serving	0	0	0	170
Scrambled Eggs	2 eggs	1	1	0	160
Hash Browns	1 serving	14	13	1	130

FAST FOOD AND OTHER RESTAURANTS

FOOD	SERVING	TOTAL CARBS (G)	NET CARBS (G)	FIBER (G)	CALORIES
Warm Cinnamon Roll	1 roll	60	58	2	440
Deluxe Warm Cinnamon Roll	1 roll	81	77	4	510
SONIC					
Sonic Bacon Egg & Cheese Toaster	1 serving	40	38	2	500
Sonic Sausage Egg & Cheese Toaster	1 serving	44	42	2	570
Sonic Ham Egg & Cheese Toaster	1 serving	41	39	2	436
Breakfast Burrito	1 serving	45	42	3	616
Sonic Sunrise, Regular	1 serving	60	59	1	224
Sonic Sunrise, Large	1 serving	100	98	2	368
SUBWAY					
Cheese & Egg Breakfast Sandwich on Deli Round	1 sandwich	34	31	3	320
Bacon & Egg Breakfast Sandwich on Deli Round	1 sandwich	34	31	3	320
Western & Egg Breakfast Sandwich on Deli Round	1 sandwich	36	33	3	300
Steak & Egg Breakfast Sandwich on Deli Round	1 sandwich	35	32	3	330
Ham & Egg Breakfast Sandwich on Deli Round	1 sandwich	34	31	3	310

FAST FOOD AND OTHER RESTAURANTS

FOOD	SERVING	TOTAL CARBS (G)	NET CARBS (G)	FIBER (G)	CALORIES
Vegetable & Egg Breakfast Sandwich on Deli Round	1 sandwich	36	33	3	290
Cheese & Egg Breakfast Sandwich (on Italian or Wheat Bread)	6" sub sandwich	42	39	3	440
Bacon & Egg Breakfast Sandwich (on Italian or Wheat Bread)	6" sub sandwich	42	39	3	450
Western & Egg Breakfast Sandwich (on Italian or Wheat Bread)	6" sub sandwich	44	40	4	430
Steak & Egg Breakfast Sandwich (on Italian or Wheat Bread)	6" sub sandwich	43	39	4	460
Ham & Egg Breakfast Sandwich (on Italian or Wheat Bread)	6" sub sandwich	42	39	3	430
Vegetable & Egg Breakfast Sandwich (on Italian or Wheat Bread)	6" sub sandwich	44	40	4	410
Cheese & Egg Omelet	1 omelet	2	2	0	240
Bacon & Egg Omelet	1 omelet	2	2	0	240
Western & Egg Omelet	1 omelet	4	3	1	220
Steak & Egg Omelet	1 omelet	3	2	1	250
Ham & Egg Omelet	1 omelet	2	2	0	230
Vegetable & Egg Omelet	1 omelet	4	3	1	210
French Toast w/Syrup	1 serving	57	55	2	350

CHICKEN AND CHICKEN ITEMS

HARDEE'S

FOOD	SERVING	TOTAL CARBS (G)	NET CARBS (G)	FIBER (G)	CALORIES
Chicken Strips (3)	3 strips	27	26	1	380
Chicken Strips (5)	5 strips	45	43	2	630
Chicken Strips, Kids Meal, w/o sauce	1 meal	50	47	3	500
Fried Chicken Breast	1 breast	29	29	0	370
Fried Chicken Wing	1 wing	23	23	0	200
Fried Chicken Thigh	1 thigh	30	30	0	330
Fried Chicken Leg	1 leg	15	15	0	170

JACK IN THE BOX

FOOD	SERVING	TOTAL CARBS (G)	NET CARBS (G)	FIBER (G)	CALORIES
Chicken Breast Strips	1 serving	39	36	3	630

KFC (KENTUCKY FRIED CHICKEN)

FOOD	SERVING	TOTAL CARBS (G)	NET CARBS (G)	FIBER (G)	CALORIES
Original Recipe, Whole Wing	1 wing	5	5	0	150
Original Recipe, Breast	1 breast	11	11	0	380
Original Recipe, Breast w/o Skin or Breading	1 breast	0	0	0	140
Original Recipe, Drumstick	1 drumstick	4	4	0	140
Original Recipe, Thigh	1 thigh	12	12	0	360
Extra Crispy, Whole Wing	1 wing	10	10	0	190
Extra Crispy, Breast	1 breast	19	19	0	460
Extra Crispy, Drumstick	1 drumstick	5	5	0	160
Extra Crispy, Thigh	1 thigh	12	12	0	370
Hot & Spicy Chicken, Whole Wing	1 wing	9	9	0	180
Hot & Spicy Chicken, Breast	1 breast	20	20	0	460

FOOD	SERVING	TOTAL CARBS (G)	NET CARBS (G)	FIBER (G)	CALORIES
Hot & Spicy Chicken, Drumstick	1 drumstick	4	4	0	150
Hot & Spicy Chicken, Thigh	1 thigh	14	14	0	400
Crispy Strips	3 strips	17	17	0	400
Popcorn Chicken for Kids	1 serving	16	16	0	270
Popcorn Chicken for Individual	1 serving	25	25	0	450
Popcorn Chicken, Large	1 serving	37	37	0	660
Chicken Pot Pie	1 pie	70	65	5	770
Hot BBQ Boneless Wings, sauced	7 wings	49	47	2	600
Hot BBQ Wings, sauced	6 wings	36	35	1	540
Hot Wings	6 wings	23	22	1	450
LONG JOHN SILVER'S					
Battered Chicken	1 piece	9	9	0	140
MCDONALD'S					
Chicken McNuggets, Made w/White Meat	4 pieces	10	10	0	170
Chicken McNuggets, Made w/White Meat	6 pieces	15	15	0	250
Chicken McNuggets, Made w/White Meat	10 pieces	26	26	0	420
Chicken McNuggets, Made w/White Meat	20 pieces	51	51	0	840
SONIC					
Chicken Strip Dinner	1 dinner	86	81	5	749
Chicken Strip Snack	1 serving	22	22	0	272

138 FAST FOOD AND OTHER RESTAURANTS

FOOD	SERVING	TOTAL CARBS (G)	NET CARBS (G)	FIBER (G)	CALORIES
WENDY'S					
Homestyle Chicken Strips	3 strips	33	33	0	410
Chicken Nuggets, 4 Piece Kids' Meal	4 pieces	10	10	0	180
Chicken Nuggets, 5 Pieces	5 pieces	13	13	0	220
DESSERTS					
ARBY'S					
Apple Turnover, Iced	1 turnover (4.5 oz)	65	63	2	420
Cherry Turnover, Iced	1 turnover (4.5 oz)	63	62	1	410
BLIMPIE					
Chocolate Chunk Cookie	1 cookie	26	25	1	200
Macadamia White Chunk Cookie	1 cookie	26	25	1	210
Oatmeal Raisin Cookie	1 cookie	27	26	1	190
Peanut Butter Cookie	1 cookie	23	22	1	220
Sugar Cookie	1 cookie	24.2	24.2	0	330
BURGER KING					
Dutch Apple Pie	1 pie (113 g)	52	51	1	340
Hershey's Sundae Pie	1 pie (79 g)	31	30	1	300
Nestlé Toll House Freshly Baked Chocolate Chip Cookies	2 cookies (96 g)	68	68	0	440
CHICK-FIL-A					
Icedream	1 small cup (7.5 g)	38	38	0	230
Icedream	1 small cone (4.7 g)	28	28	0	160
Lemon Pie	1 slice (4 g)	51	48	3	320

FAST FOOD AND OTHER RESTAURANTS

FOOD	SERVING	TOTAL CARBS (G)	NET CARBS (G)	FIBER (G)	CALORIES
Fudge Nut Brownie	1 brownie (2.6 g)	45	43	2	330
Cheesecake	1 slice (3.3 g)	30	28	2	340
Cheesecake w/ Strawberry Topping	1 slice (4.1 g)	38	36	2	360
Cheesecake w/ Blueberry Topping	1 slice (4.1 g)	39	37	2	370
DENNY'S					
Apple Pie	1 serving	64	63	1	470
Coconut Cream Pie	1 serving	63	60	3	582
French Silk Pie	1 serving	54	50	4	690
Apple Crisp à la mode	1 serving	133	127	6	723
Chocolate Peanut Butter Pie	1 serving	64	61	3	653
Cheesecake	1 serving	51	51	0	580
Carrot Cake	1 serving	99	97	2	799
Hot Fudge Brownie à la mode	1 serving	147	141	6	997
Hot Fudge Brownie for Kids	1 serving	49	47	2	344
Banana Split	1 serving	121	115	6	894
Double Scoop Sundae	1 serving	29	29	0	375
Single Scoop Sundae	1 serving	14	14	0	188
HARDEE'S					
Chocolate Chip Cookie	1 cookie	44	44	0	290
Apple Turnover	1 turnover	36	35	1	290
JACK IN THE BOX					
Cheesecake	1 serving	34	34	0	310
Double Fudge Cake	1 serving	49	45	4	310

FOOD	SERVING	TOTAL CARBS (G)	NET CARBS (G)	FIBER (G)	CALORIES
KFC (KENTUCKY FRIED CHICKEN)					
Double Chocolate Chip Cookie	1 cookie	31	29	2	400
Lil' Bucket Fudge Brownie	1 brownie	44	43	1	270
Lil' Bucket Lemon Crème	1 serving	65	63	2	400
Lil' Bucket Chocolate Crème	1 serving	37	35	2	270
Strawberry Crème Pie Slice	1 slice	37	37	0	270
Lil' Bucket Strawberry Shortcake	1 serving	34	34	0	200
Pecan Pie Slice	1 slice	55	53	2	370
Apple Pie Slice	1 slice	45	41	4	270
Lemon Meringue Pie	1 slice	47	44	3	310
Cherry Cheesecake Parfait	1 serving	46	44	2	300
LONG JOHN SILVER'S					
Chocolate Cream Pie	1 pie	24	23	1	310
Pineapple Cream Pie	1 pie	39	38	1	290
Pecan Pie	1 pie	55	53	2	370
MCDONALD'S					
Fruit 'n Yogurt Parfait	1 serving	30	30	t	160
Fruit 'n Yogurt Parfait w/o Granola	1 serving	25	25	0	130
Apple Dippers w/Low Fat Caramel Dip	1 serving	22	22	0	100
Vanilla Reduced Fat Ice Cream Cone	1 cone	23	23	0	150

FOOD	SERVING	TOTAL CARBS (G)	NET CARBS (G)	FIBER (G)	CALORIES
Kiddie Cone	1 cone	7	7	0	45
Strawberry Sundae	1 sundae	50	50	t	290
Hot Caramel Sundae	1 sundae	61	61	0	360
Hot Fudge Sundae	1 sundae	52	51	1	340
M&M McFlurry	12 fl oz	90	98	1	630
Oreo McFlurry	12 fl oz	82	82	t	570
Baked Apple Pie	1 pie	34	34	t	260
McDonaldland Chocolate Chip Cookies	1 serving	37	36	1	280
McDonaldland Cookies	1 serving	38	38	1	230
Chocolate Chip Cookie	1 cookie	22	22	t	160
Oatmeal Raisin Cookie	1 cookie	23	22	1	150
Sugar Cookie	1 cookie	20	20	0	140
PIZZA HUT					
Cinnamon Sticks	2 sticks	27	27	t	170
White Icing Dipping Cup	1 serving (2 oz)	46	46	0	190
Apple Dessert Pizza	1 slice	53	52	2	260
Cherry Dessert Pizza	1 slice	47	46	1	240
RUBY TUESDAY					
Chocolate Tallcake	1 serving	na	106	0	756
Chocolate Shortcake	1 serving	na	90	0	636
Low Carb Cheesecake	1 serving	na	6	1	360
Strawberry Tallcake	1 serving	na	80	1	583
Strawberry Shortcake	1 serving	na	53	1	428
Blondie	1 serving	na	102	2	745
Blueberry D'lite	1 serving	na	34	4	214
SCHLOTZSKY'S DELI					
Chocolate Chip Cookie	1 serving	23	23	0	160

142 FAST FOOD AND OTHER RESTAURANTS

FOOD	SERVING	TOTAL CARBS (G)	NET CARBS (G)	FIBER (G)	CALORIES
Oatmeal Raisin Cookie	1 serving	24	23	1	150
Peanut Butter Cookie	1 serving	21	20	1	170
Sugar Cookie	1 serving	23	23	0	160
White Chocolate Macadamia Cookie	1 serving	22	22	0	170
Fudge Chocolate Chip Cookie	1 serving	22	21	1	170
Cranberry Walnut Crunch Cookie	1 serving	23	22	1	160
Golden Raisin Oatmeal Cookie	1 serving	23	22	1	160
Triple Chocolate Chip Cookie	1 serving	21	20	1	170
Cookies w/Real M&M's	1 serving	20	20	0	140
New York Creamstyle Cheesecake	1 serving	31	31	0	310
Strawberry Swirl Cheesecake	1 serving	30	30	0	300
Cookies & Crème Cheesecake	1 serving	36	35	1	330
Fudge Brownie Cake	1 serving	46	43	3	410
SONIC					
Banana Split	1 serving	75	72	3	467
Hot Fudge Sundae	1 serving	40	40	0	392
Strawberry Sundae	1 serving	32	31	1	322
Chocolate Sundae	1 serving	41	41	0	362
Pineapple Sundae	1 serving	53	53	0	399
Ice Cream Cone	1 serving	23	32	0	285
Dish of Vanilla	1 serving	19	19	0	265

FOOD	SERVING	TOTAL CARBS (G)	NET CARBS (G)	FIBER (G)	CALORIES
SUBWAY					
Chocolate Chip Cookie	1 cookie	30	29	1	210
Oatmeal Raisin Cookie	1 cookie	30	28	2	200
Peanut Butter Cookie	1 cookie	26	25	1	220
M&M Cookie	1 cookie	30	29	1	210
White Macadamia Nut Cookie	1 cookie	28	27	1	220
Sugar Cookie	1 cookie	28	28	0	230
Chocolate Chunk Cookie	1 cookie	30	29	1	220
Double Chocolate Chip Cookie	1 cookie	30	29	1	210
Atkins-Friendly Double Chocolate Cookie	1 cookie	17	7	5	100
Apple Pie	1 pie	37	36	1	245
Fruit Roll-Up	1 roll-up	12	12	0	50
TCBY					
Nonfat Frozen Yogurt	½ cup (98 g)	23	23	0	110
Nonfat Frozen Yogurt, No Sugar Added	½ cup (96 g)	20	20	0	80
96% Fat Free Frozen Yogurt	½ cup (97 g)	23	23	0	130
Nonfat & Nondairy Sorbet	½ cup (97 g)	24	24	0	100
Vanilla Low Carb Lovers	½ cup (92 g)	17	10	7	110
Chocolate Low Carb Lovers	½ cup (92 g)	17	10	7	110

144 FAST FOOD AND OTHER RESTAURANTS

FOOD	SERVING	TOTAL CARBS (G)	NET CARBS (G)	FIBER (G)	CALORIES
DINNER ENTRÉES					
CHILI'S					
Grill Platters, Monterey Chicken w/Veggies, w/o Garlic Bread	1 order	24	18	6	951
Grill Platters, Ribeye w/Veggies, w/o Garlic Bread	1 order	8	4	4	907
Grill Platters, Salmon w/Veggies, w/o Garlic Bread	1 order	11	7	4	412
Guiltless Grill Chicken Platter	1 platter	83	79	4	563
Guiltless Grill Tomato Basil Pasta Platter	1 platter	106	106	0	671
Knife & Fork Fajitas, Beef w/Veggies, Sour Cream, Pico de Gallo & Guacamole, w/o Tortilla	1 order	17	7	10	647
Knife & Fork Fajitas, Beef/Chicken Combo w/Veggies, Sour Cream, Pico de Gallo & Guacamole, w/o Tortilla	1 order	17	7	10	600

FOOD	SERVING	TOTAL CARBS (G)	NET CARBS (G)	FIBER (G)	CALORIES
Knife & Fork Fajitas, Chicken w/Veggies, Sour Cream, Pico de Gallo & Guacamole, w/o Tortilla	1 order	17	7	10	432
Knife & Fork Fajitas, Mushroom Jack w/Veggies, Sour Cream, Pico de Gallo & Guacamole, w/o Tortilla	1 order	24	13	11	978

DENNY'S

FOOD	SERVING	TOTAL CARBS (G)	NET CARBS (G)	FIBER (G)	CALORIES
Carb-Watch T-bone	1 serving	8	5	3	791
Carb-Watch Sirloin Steak	1 serving	8	5	3	368
Carb-Watch Grilled Chicken Dinner	1 serving	8	5	3	314
Carb-Watch Roast Turkey Dinner	1 serving	11	8	3	379
T-bone Steak Dinner*	1 serving	0	0	0	860
Sirloin Steak Dinner*	1 serving	1	0	1	337
Pot Roast Dinner*	1 serving	5	5	0	292
Country Fried Steak*	1 serving	30	19	11	644
Fried Shrimp & Scrimp Scampi*	1 serving	15	16	1	346
Steak & Shrimp Dinner*	1 serving	31	29	2	645
Fried Shrimp Dinner*	1 serving	18	17	1	219

* Side dishes not included in nutrient count. See section on "Side Items and Other Individual Items: Denny's" (p. 196) for side dish nutrient count.

FAST FOOD AND OTHER RESTAURANTS

FOOD	SERVING	TOTAL CARBS (G)	NET CARBS (G)	FIBER (G)	CALORIES
Roast Turkey & Stuffing, Gravy Included*	1 serving	62	60	2	435
Shrimp Scampi Skillet Dinner*	1 serving	3	2.7	.3	289
Grilled Chicken Dinner*	1 serving	15	14	1	200
Fish & Chips	1 serving	83	57	6	958
Chicken Strips*	1 serving	55	55	0	635
Fisherman's Platter	1 serving	89	79	10	1,027
O'CHARLEY'S (LOW CARB MENU)					
10 oz Flame Grilled Sirloin w/Side Item & House Salad[†]	1 dinner	na	5.5	na	na
7 oz Flame Grilled Sirloin w/Side Item & House Salad[†]	1 dinner	na	5.5	na	na
Bacon Cheese Chicken Trio w/Side Item[†]	1 dinner	na	4	na	na
Chicken Cordon Bleu w/Side Item[†]	1 dinner	na	5	na	na
9 oz Filet Mignon w/Side Item[†]	1 dinner	na	2	na	na
Fresh Atlantic Salmon w/Side Item & House Salad[†]	1 dinner	na	5.25	na	na
Prime Time Prime Rib w/Side Item & House Salad[†]	1 dinner	na	5.5	na	na

* Side dishes not included in nutrient count. See section on "Side Items and Other Individual Items: Denny's" (p. 196) for side dish nutrient count.
[†] Net carbs included only for meat/fish entrée; side item or salad not included in nutrient count.

FAST FOOD AND OTHER RESTAURANTS

FOOD	SERVING	TOTAL CARBS (G)	NET CARBS (G)	FIBER (G)	CALORIES
Ribeye Steak w/Side Item & House Salad*	1 dinner	na	5.5	na	na
RUBY TUESDAY					
Buffalo Tenders Platter	1 serving	na	71	6	1,108
Chicken Parmesan w/Pasta	1 serving	na	70	6	1,275
Chicken Tenders Platter	1 serving	na	66	6	883
Church Street Chicken	1 serving	na	35	9	687
Church Street Chicken, Low Carb	1 serving	na	12	12	659
Creole Catch	1 serving	na	34	6	543
Creole Catch, Low Carb	1 serving	na	11	10	515
Stacked Steak	1 serving	na	63	10	1,346
Chopped Steak, Low Carb	1 serving	na	11	10	625
Glazed Peppercorn Chilean Salmon	1 serving	na	43	10	661
Glazed Peppercorn Chilean Salmon, Low Carb	1 serving	na	19	10	535
"Hang off the Plate" Ribs, Half Rack	1 half rack	na	57	6	944
"Hang off the Plate" Ribs, Full Rack	1 full rack	na	72	6	1,437
Louisiana Fried Shrimp	1 serving	na	87	7	1,006
Memphis Ribs, Half Rack	1 half rack	na	46	6	989
Memphis Ribs, Full Rack	1 full rack	na	50	6	1,527

* Net carbs included only for meat/fish entrée; side item or salad not included in nutrient count.

FAST FOOD AND OTHER RESTAURANTS

FOOD	SERVING	TOTAL CARBS (G)	NET CARBS (G)	FIBER (G)	CALORIES
New Orleans Seafood	1 serving	na	37	6	739
Pasta Marinara	1 serving	na	81	8	514
Pepper Bleu Steak	1 serving	na	4	0	471
Peppercorn Mushroom Sirloin Steak	1 serving	na	6	2	613
Petite Sirloin Steak	1 serving	na	1	0	222
Roasted Turkey & Gravy Dinner	1 serving	na	34	10	605
Roasted Turkey & Gravy Dinner, Low Carb	1 serving	na	14	10	628
Roma Chicken Alfredo Pasta	1 serving	na	79	8	928
Ruby's Ribeye Steak	1 serving	na	4	0	635
Shrimp Alfredo Pasta	1 serving	na	78	8	896
Shrimp Azteca	1 serving	na	101	8	810
Sirloin Tips, Half Rack	1 half rack	na	6	0	390
Sirloin Tips, Full Rack	1 full rack	na	7	0	611
Smoky Mountain Chicken	1 serving	na	49	7	692
Sonora Chicken Pasta	1 serving	na	89	11	966
Spicy Honey BBQ Ribs, Half Rack	1 half rack	na	62	6	959
Spicy Honey BBQ Ribs, Full Rack	1 full rack	na	81	6	1,467
Spicy Honey BBQ Ribeye Steak	1 serving	na	24	0	715
Spicy Honey BBQ Tenders Platter	1 serving	na	96	6	1,003
Steak & Shrimp Remoulade	1 serving	na	15	1	794

FOOD	SERVING	TOTAL CARBS (G)	NET CARBS (G)	FIBER (G)	CALORIES
Top Sirloin Steak	1 serving	na	1	0	285
Triple Play (Ribs & Tenders)	1 serving	na	93	6	1,481
Veggie Platter	1 serving	na	36	15	395
Veggie Platter, Low Carb	1 serving	na	17	14	297
T.G.I. FRIDAY'S					
Sizzling NY Strip w/Bleu Cheese, w/Side of Broccoli	1 serving	na	6	na	na
Bunless Burgers w/Small Salad of Exotic Greens	1 serving	na	6	na	na
Sizzling Chicken w/Broccoli	1 serving	na	17	na	na
Garlic Chicken w/Mixed Vegetables	1 serving	na	7	na	na
Fire Roasted Salmon Fillet	1 serving	na	12	na	na
FISH AND SEAFOOD					
LONG JOHN SILVER'S					
Battered Fish	1 piece	16	16	0	230
Baked Cod	1 piece	0	0	1	120
Battered Shrimp	1 piece	3	3	0	45
Crunchy Shrimp Basket	21 pieces	31	29	2	330
Breaded Clams	1 serving	22	21	1	240
JACK IN THE BOX					
Fish & Chips	1 serving	69	65	4	840

FAST FOOD AND OTHER RESTAURANTS

FOOD	SERVING	TOTAL CARBS (G)	NET CARBS (G)	FIBER (G)	CALORIES
PIZZAS					
DOMINO'S					
Beef, 12" Classic Hand Tossed	1 slice (⅛ of pizza)	28	26	2	225
Beef, 12" Ultimate Deep Dish	1 slice (⅛ of pizza)	28	26	2	227
Beef, 12" Crunchy Thin Crust	1 slice (⅛ of pizza)	14	14	1	175
Beef, 14" Classic Hand Tossed	1 slice (⅛ of pizza)	38	36	2	312
Beef, 14" Ultimate Deep Dish	1 slice (⅛ of pizza)	41	39	2	392
Beef, 14" Crunchy Thin Crust	1 slice (⅛ of pizza)	19	18	1	243
Cheese, 12" Classic Hand Tossed	1 slice (⅛ of pizza)	28	27	1	186
Cheese, 12" Ultimate Deep Dish	1 slice (⅛ of pizza)	28	26	2	238
Cheese, 12" Crunchy Thin Crust	1 slice (⅛ of pizza)	14	13	1	137
Cheese, 14" Classic Hand Tossed	1 slice (⅛ of pizza)	38	36	2	256
Cheese, 14" Ultimate Deep Dish	1 slice (⅛ of pizza)	41	39	2	336
Cheese, 14" Crunchy Thin Crust	1 slice (⅛ of pizza)	19	18	1	188
Deluxe Feast, 12" Classic Hand Tossed	1 slice (⅛ of pizza)	29	27	2	234
Deluxe Feast, 12" Ultimate Deep Dish	1 slice (⅛ of pizza)	29	27	2	287
Deluxe Feast, 12" Crunchy Thin Crust	1 slice (⅛ of pizza)	15	14	1	185

FAST FOOD AND OTHER RESTAURANTS 151

FOOD	SERVING	TOTAL CARBS (G)	NET CARBS (G)	FIBER (G)	CALORIES
Deluxe Feast, 14" Classic Hand Tossed	1 slice (⅛ of pizza)	39	37	2	316
Deluxe Feast, 14" Ultimate Deep Dish	1 slice (⅛ of pizza)	42	39	3	396
Deluxe Feast, 14" Crunchy Thin Crust	1 slice (⅛ of pizza)	20	18	2	248
ExtravaganZZa Feast, 12" Classic Hand Tossed	1 slice (⅛ of pizza)	30	28	2	289
ExtravaganZZa Feast, 12" Ultimate Deep Dish	1 slice (⅛ of pizza)	30	28	2	341
ExtravaganZZa Feast, 12" Crunchy Thin Crust	1 slice (⅛ of pizza)	16	15	1	240
ExtravaganZZa Feast, 14" Classic Hand Tossed	1 slice (⅛ of pizza)	40	37	3	388
ExtravaganZZa Feast, 14" Ultimate Deep Dish	1 slice (⅛ of pizza)	43	40	3	468
ExtravaganZZa Feast, 14" Crunchy Thin Crust	1 slice (⅛ of pizza)	21	19	2	320
Green Pepper, Onion & Mushroom, 12" Classic Hand Tossed	1 slice (⅛ of pizza)	29	27	2	191
Green Pepper, Onion & Mushroom, 12" Ultimate Deep Dish	1 slice (⅛ of pizza)	30	28	2	244

FOOD	SERVING	TOTAL CARBS (G)	NET CARBS (G)	FIBER (G)	CALORIES
Green Pepper, Onion & Mushroom, 12" Crunchy Thin Crust	1 slice (⅛ of pizza)	15	14	1	142
Green Pepper, Onion & Mushroom, 14" Classic Hand Tossed	1 slice (⅛ of pizza)	39	37	2	263
Green Pepper, Onion & Mushroom, 14" Ultimate Deep Dish	1 slice (⅛ of pizza)	42	39	3	343
Green Pepper, Onion & Mushroom, 14" Crunchy Thin Crust	1 slice (⅛ of pizza)	21	19	2	201
Ham, 12" Classic Hand Tossed	1 slice (⅛ of pizza)	28	27	1	198
Ham, 12" Ultimate Deep Dish	1 slice (⅛ of pizza)	28	26	2	250
Ham, 12" Crunchy Thin Crust	1 slice (⅛ of pizza)	14	13	1	148
Ham, 14" Classic Hand Tossed	1 slice (⅛ of pizza)	38	26	2	272
Ham, 14" Ultimate Deep Dish	1 slice (⅛ of pizza)	41	39	2	352
Ham, 14" Crunchy Thin Crust	1 slice (⅛ of pizza)	19	18	1	204
Ham & Pineapple, 12" Classic Hand Tossed	1 slice (⅛ of pizza)	29	27	2	200
Ham & Pineapple, 12" Ultimate Deep Dish	1 slice (⅛ of pizza)	30	28	2	252
Ham & Pineapple, 12" Crunchy Thin Crust	1 slice (⅛ of pizza)	15	14	1	150
Ham & Pineapple, 14" Classic Hand Tossed	1 slice (⅛ of pizza)	40	38	2	275

FAST FOOD AND OTHER RESTAURANTS 153

FOOD	SERVING	TOTAL CARBS (G)	NET CARBS (G)	FIBER (G)	CALORIES
Ham & Pineapple, 14" Ultimate Deep Dish	1 slice (⅛ of pizza)	42	40	2	355
Ham & Pineapple, 14" Crunchy Thin Crust	1 slice (⅛ of pizza)	21	20	1	207
Hawaiian Feast, 12" Classic Hand Tossed	1 slice (⅛ of pizza)	30	28	2	223
Hawaiian Feast, 12" Ultimate Deep Dish	1 slice (⅛ of pizza)	30	28	2	275
Hawaiian Feast, 12" Crunchy Thin Crust	1 slice (⅛ of pizza)	16	15	1	174
Hawaiian Feast, 14" Classic Hand Tossed	1 slice (⅛ of pizza)	41	39	2	309
Hawaiian Feast, 14" Ultimate Deep Dish	1 slice (⅛ of pizza)	43	40	3	389
Hawaiian Feast, 14" Crunchy Thin Crust	1 slice (⅛ of pizza)	21	19	2	240
MeatZZa Feast, 12" Classic Hand Tossed	1 slice (⅛ of pizza)	29	27	2	281
MeatZZa Feast, 12" Ultimate Deep Dish	1 slice (⅛ of pizza)	29	27	2	333
MeatZZa Feast, 12" Crunchy Thin Crust	1 slice (⅛ of pizza)	15	14	1	232
MeatZZa Feast, 14" Classic Hand Tossed	1 slice (⅛ of pizza)	39	37	2	378
MeatZZa Feast, 14" Ultimate Deep Dish	1 slice (⅛ of pizza)	42	39	3	458
MeatZZa Feast, 14" Crunchy Thin Crust	1 slice (⅛ of pizza)	20	18	2	310
Pepperoni, 12" Classic Hand Tossed	1 slice (⅛ of pizza)	28	26	2	223

FAST FOOD AND OTHER RESTAURANTS

FOOD	SERVING	TOTAL CARBS (G)	NET CARBS (G)	FIBER (G)	CALORIES
Pepperoni, 12" Ultimate Deep Dish	1 slice (⅛ of pizza)	28	26	2	275
Pepperoni, 12" Crunchy Thin Crust	1 slice (⅛ of pizza)	14	13	1	174
Pepperoni, 14" Classic Hand Tossed	1 slice (⅛ of pizza)	38	36	2	305
Pepperoni, 14" Ultimate Deep Dish	1 slice (⅛ of pizza)	41	39	2	385
Pepperoni, 14" Crunchy Thin Crust	1 slice (⅛ of pizza)	19	18	1	237
Pepperoni & Sausage, 12" Classic Hand Tossed	1 slice (⅛ of pizza)	28	26	2	255
Pepperoni & Sausage, 12" Ultimate Deep Dish	1 slice (⅛ of pizza)	29	27	2	307
Pepperoni & Sausage, 12" Crunchy Thin Crust	1 slice (⅛ of pizza)	14	13	1	206
Pepperoni & Sausage, 14" Classic Hand Tossed	1 slice (⅛ of pizza)	39	37	2	350
Pepperoni & Sausage, 14" Ultimate Deep Dish	1 slice (⅛ of pizza)	41	39	3	430
Pepperoni & Sausage, 14" Crunchy Thin Crust	1 slice (⅛ of pizza)	19	17	2	282
Pepperoni Feast, 12" Classic Hand Tossed	1 slice (⅛ of pizza)	28	26	2	265
Pepperoni Feast, 12" Ultimate Deep Dish	1 slice (⅛ of pizza)	29	27	2	317
Pepperoni Feast, 12" Crunchy Thin Crust	1 slice (⅛ of pizza)	14	13	1	216
Pepperoni Feast, 14" Classic Hand Tossed	1 slice (⅛ of pizza)	39	37	2	363
Pepperoni Feast, 14" Ultimate Deep Dish	1 slice (⅛ of pizza)	42	39	3	443

FAST FOOD AND OTHER RESTAURANTS

FOOD	SERVING	TOTAL CARBS (G)	NET CARBS (G)	FIBER (G)	CALORIES
Pepperoni Feast, 14" Crunchy Thin Crust	1 slice (⅛ of pizza)	20	19	1	295
Sausage, 12" Classic Hand Tossed	1 slice (⅛ of pizza)	28	26	2	231
Sausage, 12" Ultimate Deep Dish	1 slice (⅛ of pizza)	29	27	2	283
Sausage, 12" Crunchy Thin Crust	1 slice (⅛ of pizza)	14	13	1	181
Sausage, 14" Classic Hand Tossed	1 slice (⅛ of pizza)	39	37	2	320
Sausage, 14" Ultimate Deep Dish	1 slice (⅛ of pizza)	42	39	3	400
Sausage, 14" Crunchy Thin Crust	1 slice (⅛ of pizza)	20	18	2	252
Vegi Feast, 12" Classic Hand Tossed	1 slice (⅛ of pizza)	29	27	2	218
Vegi Feast, 12" Ultimate Deep Dish	1 slice (⅛ of pizza)	30	28	2	270
Vegi Feast, 12" Crunchy Thin Crust	1 slice (⅛ of pizza)	15	14	1	168
Vegi Feast, 14" Classic Hand Tossed	1 slice (⅛ of pizza)	40	37	3	300
Vegi Feast, 14" Ultimate Deep Dish	1 slice (⅛ of pizza)	43	40	3	380
Vegi Feast, 14" Crunchy Thin Crust	1 slice (⅛ of pizza)	21	19	2	231
PAPA JOHN'S					
Cheese, Thin Crust Pizza	1 slice (⅛ of 14" pizza)	23	22	1	238
Pepperoni, Thin Crust Pizza	1 slice (⅛ of 14" pizza)	23	21.5	1.5	294

FAST FOOD AND OTHER RESTAURANTS

FOOD	SERVING	TOTAL CARBS (G)	NET CARBS (G)	FIBER (G)	CALORIES
Sausage, Thin Crust Pizza	1 slice (⅛ of 14" pizza)	24	22.5	1.5	303
All the Meats w/Beef, Thin Crust Pizza	1 slice (⅛ of 14" pizza)	24	22.5	1.5	371
All the Meats w/o Beef, Thin Crust Pizza	1 slice (⅛ of 14" pizza)	23	22	1	109
Garden Fresh, Thin Crust Pizza	1 slice (⅛ of 14" pizza)	24	22	2	228
The Works, Thin Crust Pizza	1 slice (⅛ of 14" pizza)	25	23	2	315
Spinach Alfredo, Thin Crust Pizza	1 slice (⅛ of 14" pizza)	22	21	1	251
Chicken Alfredo, Thin Crust Pizza	1 slice (⅛ of 14" pizza)	22	21	1	276
BBQ Chicken & Bacon, Thin Crust Pizza	1 slice (⅛ of 14" pizza)	30	29	1	336
Hawaiian BBQ Chicken, Thin Crust Pizza	1 slice (⅛ of 14" pizza)	31	29.7	1.3	324
Cheese, Original Crust Pizza	1 slice (⅛ of 14" pizza)	39	37	2	290
Pepperoni, Original Crust Pizza	1 slice (⅛ of 14" pizza)	39	37	2	343
Sausage, Original Crust Pizza	1 slice (⅛ of 14" pizza)	38	36	2	336
All the Meats w/Beef, Original Crust Pizza	1 slice (⅛ of 14" pizza)	39	27	2	405
All the Meats w/o Beef, Original Crust Pizza	1 slice (⅛ of 14" pizza)	38	36	2	348
Garden Fresh, Original Crust Pizza	1 slice (⅛ of 14" pizza)	40	37	3	287

FAST FOOD AND OTHER RESTAURANTS 157

FOOD	SERVING	TOTAL CARBS (G)	NET CARBS (G)	FIBER (G)	CALORIES
The Works, Original Crust Pizza	1 slice (⅛ of 14" pizza)	40	37	3	370
Spinach Alfredo, Original Crust Pizza	1 slice (⅛ of 14" pizza)	37	35	2	303
Chicken Alfredo, Original Crust Pizza	1 slice (⅛ of 14" pizza)	37	35	2	310
BBQ Chicken & Bacon, Original Crust Pizza	1 slice (⅛ of 14" pizza)	44	42	2	369
Hawaiian BBQ Chicken, Original Crust Pizza	1 slice (⅛ of 14" pizza)	46	44	2	376
PIZZA HUT					
12" Medium Pan Pizza, Cheese Only	1 slice	29	28	1	280
12" Medium Pan Pizza, Pepperoni	1 slice	29	26	2	290
12" Medium Pan Pizza, Quartered Ham	1 slice	29	28	1	260
12" Medium Pan Pizza, Supreme	1 slice	30	28	2	320
12" Medium Pan Pizza, Super Supreme	1 slice	30	28	2	340
12" Medium Pan Pizza, Chicken Supreme	1 slice	30	28	2	280
12" Medium Pan Pizza, Meat Lover's	1 slice	29	27	2	340
12" Medium Pan Pizza, Veggie Lover's	1 slice	30	28	2	260
12" Medium Pan Pizza, Pepperoni Lover's	1 slice	29	27	2	340
12" Medium Pan Pizza, Sausage Lover's	1 slice	29	27	2	330

158 FAST FOOD AND OTHER RESTAURANTS

FOOD	SERVING	TOTAL CARBS (G)	NET CARBS (G)	FIBER (G)	CALORIES
12" Medium Thin 'N Crispy Pizza, Cheese Only	1 slice	21	20	1	200
12" Medium Thin 'N Crispy Pizza, Pepperoni	1 slice	21	20	1	210
12" Medium Thin 'N Crispy Pizza, Quartered Ham	1 slice	21	20	1	180
12" Medium Thin 'N Crispy Pizza, Supreme	1 slice	22	20	2	240
12" Medium Thin 'N Crispy Pizza, Super Supreme	1 slice	23	21	2	260
12" Medium Thin 'N Crispy Pizza, Chicken Supreme	1 slice	22	21	1	200
12" Medium Thin 'N Crispy Pizza, Meat Lover's	1 slice	21	20	2	270
12" Medium Thin 'N Crispy Pizza, Veggie Lover's	1 slice	23	21	2	180
12" Medium Thin 'N Crispy Pizza, Pepperoni Lover's	1 slice	21	19	2	260
12" Medium Thin 'N Crispy Pizza, Sausage Lover's	1 slice	21	19	2	240
12" Medium Hand-Tossed Style Pizza, Cheese Only	1 slice	30	28	2	240

FOOD	SERVING	TOTAL CARBS (G)	NET CARBS (G)	FIBER (G)	CALORIES
12" Medium Hand-Tossed Style Pizza, Pepperoni	1 slice	29	27	2	250
12" Medium Hand-Tossed Style Pizza, Quartered Ham	1 slice	29	27	2	220
12" Medium Hand-Tossed Style Pizza, Supreme	1 slice	30	28	2	270
12" Medium Hand-Tossed Style Pizza, Super Supreme	1 slice	31	29	2	300
12" Medium Hand-Tossed Style Pizza, Chicken Supreme	1 slice	30	28	2	230
12" Medium Hand-Tossed Style Pizza, Meat Lover's	1 slice	29	27	2	300
12" Medium Hand-Tossed Style Pizza, Veggie Lover's	1 slice	31	29	2	220
12" Medium Hand-Tossed Style Pizza, Pepperoni Lover's	1 slice	30	28	2	300
12" Medium Hand-Tossed Style Pizza, Sausage Lover's	1 slice	30	28	2	280
14" Large Pan Pizza, Cheese Only	1 slice	27	26	1	270
14" Large Pan Pizza, Pepperoni	1 slice	26	25	1	280

FAST FOOD AND OTHER RESTAURANTS

FOOD	SERVING	TOTAL CARBS (G)	NET CARBS (G)	FIBER (G)	CALORIES
14" Large Pan Pizza, Quartered Ham	1 slice	26	25	1	250
14" Large Pan Pizza, Supreme	1 slice	27	25	2	300
14" Large Pan Pizza, Super Supreme	1 slice	28	26	2	320
14" Large Pan Pizza, Chicken Supreme	1 slice	27	26	1	260
14" Large Pan Pizza, Meat Lover's	1 slice	27	25	2	320
14" Large Pan Pizza, Veggie Lover's	1 slice	28	26	2	250
14" Large Pan Pizza, Pepperoni Lover's	1 slice	27	25	2	330
14" Large Pan Pizza, Sausage Lover's	1 slice	27	25	2	300
14" Large Thin 'N Crispy Pizza, Cheese Only	1 slice	20	19	1	190
14" Large Thin 'N Crispy Pizza, Pepperoni	1 slice	19	18	1	200
14" Large Thin 'N Crispy Pizza, Quartered Ham	1 slice	19	18	1	170
14" Large Thin 'N Crispy Pizza, Supreme	1 slice	21	19	2	220
14" Large Thin 'N Crispy Pizza, Super Supreme	1 slice	21	19	2	240
14" Large Thin 'N Crispy Pizza, Chicken Supreme	1 slice	21	20	1	180
14" Large Thin 'N Crispy Pizza, Meat Lover's	1 slice	20	18	2	250

FOOD	SERVING	TOTAL CARBS (G)	NET CARBS (G)	FIBER (G)	CALORIES
14" Large Thin 'N Crispy Pizza, Veggie Lover's	1 slice	21	19	2	170
14" Large Thin 'N Crispy Pizza, Pepperoni Lover's	1 slice	20	19	1	250
14" Large Thin 'N Crispy Pizza, Sausage Lover's	1 slice	20	19	1	230
14" Large Hand-Tossed Style Pizza, Cheese Only	1 slice	27	26	1	220
14" Large Hand-Tossed Style Pizza, Pepperoni	1 slice	27	24	2	230
14" Large Hand-Tossed Style Pizza, Quartered Ham	1 slice	27	26	1	200
14" Large Hand-Tossed Style Pizza, Supreme	1 slice	28	26	2	250
14" Large Hand-Tossed Style Pizza, Super Supreme	1 slice	28	26	2	270
14" Large Hand-Tossed Style Pizza, Chicken Supreme	1 slice	28	26	2	210
14" Large Hand-Tossed Style Pizza, Meat Lover's	1 slice	27	25	2	280
14" Large Hand-Tossed Style Pizza, Veggie Lover's	1 slice	28	26	2	200
14" Large Hand-Tossed Style Pizza, Pepperoni Lover's	1 slice	27	25	2	280

162 FAST FOOD AND OTHER RESTAURANTS

FOOD	SERVING	TOTAL CARBS (G)	NET CARBS (G)	FIBER (G)	CALORIES
14" Large Hand-Tossed Style Pizza, Sausage Lover's	1 slice	27	25	2	260
14" Stuffed Crust Pizza, Cheese Only	1 slice	43	41	2	360
14" Stuffed Crust Pizza, Pepperoni	1 slice	42	39	3	370
14" Stuffed Crust Pizza, Quartered Ham	1 slice	42	40	2	340
14" Stuffed Crust Pizza, Supreme	1 slice	44	41	3	400
14" Stuffed Crust Pizza, Super Supreme	1 slice	45	42	3	440
14" Stuffed Crust Pizza, Chicken Supreme	1 slice	44	41	3	380
14" Stuffed Crust Pizza, Meat Lover's	1 slice	43	40	3	450
14" Stuffed Crust Pizza, Veggie Lover's	1 slice	45	42	3	360
14" Stuffed Crust Pizza, Pepperoni Lover's	1 slice	43	40	3	420
14" Stuffed Crust Pizza, Sausage Lover's	1 slice	43	40	3	430
16" Extra Large Pizza, Cheese Only	1 slice	51	48	3	420
16" Extra Large Pizza, Pepperoni	1 slice	50	47	3	430
16" Extra Large Pizza, Quartered Ham	1 slice	50	47	3	380
16" Extra Large Pizza, Supreme	1 slice	52	48	4	460

FAST FOOD AND OTHER RESTAURANTS 163

FOOD	SERVING	TOTAL CARBS (G)	NET CARBS (G)	FIBER (G)	CALORIES
16" Extra Large Pizza, Super Supreme	1 slice	53	49	4	490
16" Extra Large Pizza, Chicken Supreme	1 slice	52	49	3	400
16" Extra Large Pizza, Meat Lover's	1 slice	51	48	3	500
16" Extra Large Pizza, Veggie Lover's	1 slice	53	49	4	390
16" Extra Large Pizza, Pepperoni Lover's	1 slice	51	48	3	520
16" Extra Large Pizza, Sausage Lover's	1 slice	51	49	2	510
6" Personal Pan Pizza, Cheese Only	1 slice	18	18	t	160
6" Personal Pan Pizza, Pepperoni	1 slice	18	18	t	170
6" Personal Pan Pizza, Quartered Ham	1 slice	18	18	t	150
6" Personal Pan Pizza, Supreme	1 slice	19	18	1	190
6" Personal Pan Pizza, Super Supreme	1 slice	19	18	1	200
6" Personal Pan Pizza, Chicken Supreme	1 slice	19	19	t	160
6" Personal Pan Pizza, Meat Lover's	1 slice	18	17	1	200
6" Personal Pan Pizza, Veggie Lover's	1 slice	19	18	1	150
6" Personal Pan Pizza, Pepperoni Lover's	1 slice	18	17	1	200

FAST FOOD AND OTHER RESTAURANTS

FOOD	SERVING	TOTAL CARBS (G)	NET CARBS (G)	FIBER (G)	CALORIES
6" Personal Pan Pizza, Sausage Lover's	1 slice	18	17	1	190
Fit N' Delicious 12" Medium Pizza, Diced Chicken, Red Onion & Green Pepper	1 slice	23	21	2	170
Fit N' Delicious 12" Medium Pizza, Diced Chicken, Mushroom & Jalapeño	1 slice	22	20	2	170
Fit N' Delicious 12" Medium Pizza, Ham, Red Onion & Mushroom	1 slice	22	20	2	160
Fit N' Delicious 12" Medium Pizza, Ham, Pineapple & Diced Red Tomato	1 slice	24	22	2	160
Fit N' Delicious 12" Medium Pizza, Green Pepper, Red Onion & Diced Red Tomato	1 slice	24	22	2	150
Fit N' Delicious 12" Medium Pizza, Tomato, Mushroom & Jalapeño	1 slice	22	20	2	150
Fit N' Delicious 14" Large Pizza, Diced Chicken, Red Onion & Green Pepper	1 slice	22	20	2	160
Fit N' Delicious 14" Large Pizza, Diced Chicken, Mushroom & Jalapeño	1 slice	20	18	2	160

FAST FOOD AND OTHER RESTAURANTS 165

FOOD	SERVING	TOTAL CARBS (G)	NET CARBS (G)	FIBER (G)	CALORIES
Fit N' Delicious 14" Large Pizza, Ham, Red Onion & Mushroom	1 slice	21	19	2	150
Fit N' Delicious 14" Large Pizza, Ham, Pineapple & Diced Red Tomato	1 slice	22	21	1	150
Fit N' Delicious 14" Large Pizza, Green Pepper, Red Onion & Diced Red Tomato	1 slice	22	20	2	140
Fit N' Delicious 14" Large Pizza, Tomato, Mushroom & Jalapeño	1 slice	21	19	2	140
P'Zone, Pepperoni	½ P'Zone	69	66	3	610
P'Zone, Classic	½ P'Zone	71	68	3	610
P'Zone, Meat Lover's	½ P'Zone	70	67	3	680
Marinara Dipping Sauce for P'Zone	1 serving	9	7	2	45

SCHLOTZSKY'S DELI

FOOD	SERVING	TOTAL CARBS (G)	NET CARBS (G)	FIBER (G)	CALORIES
Double Cheese & Pepperoni, 8" Sourdough Pizza	1 whole pizza	77	73	4	721
Barbeque Chicken, 8" Sourdough Pizza	1 whole pizza	93	91	2	683
Vegetarian Special, 8" Sourdough Pizza	1 whole pizza	76	72	4	551
Thai Chicken, 8" Sourdough Pizza	1 whole pizza	89	84	5	663

FOOD	SERVING	TOTAL CARBS (G)	NET CARBS (G)	FIBER (G)	CALORIES
The Original Combination, 8" Sourdough Pizza	1 whole pizza	79	74	5	625
Tuscan Herb, 8" Sourdough Pizza	1 whole pizza	80	75	5	541
Three Meat, 8" Sourdough Pizza	1 whole pizza	74	71	3	805
Kung Pao, 8" Sourdough Pizza	1 whole pizza	92	87	5	718
Chicken & Pesto, 8" Sourdough Pizza	1 whole pizza	78	74	4	649
Smoked Turkey & Jalapeño, 8" Sourdough Pizza	1 whole pizza	80	76	4	624
Double Cheese, 8" Sourdough Pizza	1 whole pizza	76	72	4	580
Bacon, Tomato & Mushroom, 8" Sourdough Pizza	1 whole pizza	78	74	4	611
Fresh Tomato & Pesto, 8" Sourdough Pizza	1 whole pizza	76	72	4	539
Mediterranean, 8" Sourdough Pizza	1 whole pizza	72	69	3	524
Kid's Cheese Pizza	1 whole pizza	72	69	4	721
Kid's Pepperoni Pizza	1 whole pizza	72	69	4	507

SALADS

ARBY'S

| Caesar Salad* | 1 serving | 8 | 5 | 3 | 90 |

* Dressing not included in nutrient counts.

FOOD	SERVING	TOTAL CARBS (G)	NET CARBS (G)	FIBER (G)	CALORIES
Caesar Side Salad*	1 serving	4	2	2	45
Chicken Finger Salad*	1 serving	39	36	3	570
Grilled Chicken Caesar Salad*	1 serving	8	5	3	230
Turkey Club Salad*	1 serving	9	6	3	350
Martha's Vineyard Salad†	1 serving	22	18	4	280
Sliced Almonds for Martha's Vineyard Salad†	1 serving	2	1	1	81
Raspberry Vinaigrette for Martha's Vineyard Salad†	1 serving	16	16	0	172
Santa Fe Salad†	1 serving	40	35	5	520
Seasoned Tortilla Chips for Santa Fe Salad†	1 serving	10	9.5	.5	61
Asian Sesame Salad†	1 serving	14	11	3	170
Asian Noodles for Asian Sesame Salad†	1 serving	8	7	1	71
Sliced Almonds for Asian Sesame Salad†	1 serving	2	1	1	81
Asian Sesame Dressing†	1 serving	15	15	0	190
Garden Side Salad†	1 serving	7	4	3	35
Light Buttermilk Ranch Dressing†	1 serving	12	11	1	100
Light Vinaigrette†	1 serving	13	13	0	110
Fat Free Italian†	1 serving	7	7	0	30

* Dressing not included in nutrient counts.
† Limited Time Only items: these items may only be available at participating Arby's franchises.

168 FAST FOOD AND OTHER RESTAURANTS

FOOD	SERVING	TOTAL CARBS (G)	NET CARBS (G)	FIBER (G)	CALORIES
BLIMPIE					
Antipasto	1 salad, regular	10	7.3	2.7	244
Chef	1 salad, regular	9	6	3	212
Grilled Chicken w/Caesar Dressing	1 salad, regular	8.6	6	2.6	347
Seafood	1 salad, regular	16	12.8	3.2	122
Tuna	1 salad, regular	8	5.3	2.7	261
Zesto Pesto Turkey	1 salad, regular	31	31	0	370
Chili Ole	1 salad, regular	42	39	3	480
Roast Beef 'n Bleu	1 salad, regular	29	29	0	390
Buffalo Chicken Salad, w/Bleu Cheese Dressing (from Blimpie Carb Counter Menu)	1 salad, regular	na	5	na	na
Sicilian Salad, w/Light Italian Dressing (from Blimpie Carb Counter Menu)	1 salad, regular	na	7	na	na
BURGER KING					
Side Garden Salad w/o Dressing	1 salad (106 g)	4	4	t	20
Fire-Grilled Chicken Caesar Salad w/o Dressing or Toast	1 salad (286 g)	9	8	1	190
Fire-Grilled Shrimp Caesar Salad w/o Dressing or Toast	1 salad (291 g)	9	7	2	180
Fire-Grilled Chicken Garden Salad w/o Dressing or Toast	1 salad (344 g)	12	10	2	210

FAST FOOD AND OTHER RESTAURANTS

FOOD	SERVING	TOTAL CARBS (G)	NET CARBS (G)	FIBER (G)	CALORIES
Fire-Grilled Shrimp Garden Salad w/o Dressing or Toast	1 salad (349 g)	13	10	3	200
CHICK-FIL-A					
Chick-fil-A Chargrilled Chicken Garden Salad	1 salad (9.7 g)	9	6	3	180
Chick-fil-A Southwest Chargrilled Salad	1 salad (10.7 g)	17	12	5	240
Chick-fil-A Chick-N-Strips Salad	1 salad (11 g)	22	18	4	390
CHILI'S					
Dinner Salad, Low Carb w/Ranch Dressing, w/o Croutons	1 salad	8	5	3	319
Dinner Salad, Low Carb w/Avocado Ranch Dressing, w/o Croutons	1 salad	8	5	3	297
Dinner Salad, Low Carb w/Blue Cheese Dressing, w/o Croutons	1 salad	8	5	3	436
Fajita Beef Caesar Salad, Low Carb w/Caesar Dressing, w/o Croutons	1 salad	11	7	4	606
Fajita Chicken Caesar Salad, Low Carb w/Caesar Dressing, w/o Croutons	1 salad	11	7	4	516

FAST FOOD AND OTHER RESTAURANTS

FOOD	SERVING	TOTAL CARBS (G)	NET CARBS (G)	FIBER (G)	CALORIES
DAIRY QUEEN					
Crispy Chicken Salad w/o Dressing	1 serving	21	15	6	350
Grilled Chicken Salad w/o Dressing	1 serving	12	8	4	240
Grilled Chicken Salad w/Fat-Free Italian Dressing	1 serving	13	11	3	230
DENNY'S					
Carb-Watch Grilled Chicken Salad	1 salad	10	6	4	289
Grilled Chicken Caesar w/Dressing	1 salad	19	15	4	60
Grilled Chicken Breast Salad w/o Dressing	1 salad	10	6	4	264
Turkey Breast Salad w/o Dressing	1 salad	12	8	4	248
Fried Chicken Strip Salad w/o Dressing	1 salad	26	22	4	438
Coleslaw	1 salad	14	12	2	274
Side Caesar w/Dressing	1 salad	20	17	3	362
Side Garden Salad w/o Dressing	1 salad	6	4	2	113
JACK IN THE BOX					
Asian Chicken Salad	1 serving	58	50	8	595
Chicken Club Salad	1 serving	34	29	5	825
Greek Salad	1 serving	32	29	3	690
Side Salad	1 serving	16	16	0	155
Southwest Chicken Salad	1 serving	46	42	4	735

FOOD	SERVING	TOTAL CARBS (G)	NET CARBS (G)	FIBER (G)	CALORIES
MCDONALD'S					
Bacon Ranch Salad w/o Chicken	1 serving	7	4	3	130
California Cobb, w/o Chicken	1 serving	7	4	3	150
Caesar Salad, w/o Chicken	1 serving	7	4	3	90
Crispy Chicken Bacon Ranch Salad	1 serving	20	17	3	370
Crispy Chicken California Cobb Salad	1 serving	20	17	3	380
Fiesta Salad w/Sour Cream & Salsa	1 serving	28	23	5	450
Fiesta Salad w/salsa	1 serving	26	21	5	390
Fiesta Salad w/Sour Cream	1 serving	21	17	4	420
Fiesta Salad w/o Sour Cream & Salsa	1 serving	19	15	4	360
Grilled Chicken Bacon Ranch Salad	1 serving	9	6	3	250
Grilled Chicken Caesar Salad	1 serving	9	6	3	200
Grilled Chicken California Cobb Salad	1 serving	9	6	3	270
Side Salad	1 serving	3	2	1	15
RUBY TUESDAY					
Buffalo Chicken Salad	1 salad	na	25	4	614
Cajun Chicken Salad, Low Carb	1 salad	na	9	5	398
Carolina Chicken Salad	1 salad	na	23	5	507

FAST FOOD AND OTHER RESTAURANTS

FOOD	SERVING	TOTAL CARBS (G)	NET CARBS (G)	FIBER (G)	CALORIES
Peppercorn Chicken Caesar, Low Carb	1 salad	na	17	4	537
Spring Chicken Salad, Low Carb	1 salad	na	7	4	509
Spring Mix Salad	1 salad	na	3	2	39
SCHLOTZSKY'S DELI					
Chicken Caesar, Leaf Salad*	1 salad	4	2	2	11
Caesar, Leaf Salad*	1 salad	3	1	2	30
Smoked Turkey Chef's, Leaf Salad*	1 salad	13	10	3	199
Chinese Chicken, Leaf Salad*	1 salad	10	8	2	127
Greek, Leaf Salad*	1 salad	10	6	4	158
Garden, Leaf Salad*	1 salad	7	4	3	48
Small Garden, Leaf Salad*	1 salad	3	1	2	23
Ham & Turkey Chef's, Leaf Salad*	1 salad	13	10	3	202
Chow Mein Noodles	1 serving	9	8	1	74
Garlic Cheese Croutons	1 serving	5	5	0	46
Albacore Tuna, Deli Salad, Small	1 salad	2	2	0	136
Albacore Tuna, Deli Salad	1 salad	8	5	3	218
California Pasta, Deli Salad	1 salad (5 oz)	10	9	1	58
Chicken, Deli Salad, Small	1 salad	6	4	2	286

* Does not include salad dressing, croutons, or chow mein noodles.

FAST FOOD AND OTHER RESTAURANTS

FOOD	SERVING	TOTAL CARBS (G)	NET CARBS (G)	FIBER (G)	CALORIES
Chicken, Deli Salad	1 salad	13	8	5	376
Chicken & Pesto Pasta, Deli Salad, Small	1 salad	40	37	3	326
Chicken & Pesto Pasta, Deli Salad	1 salad	55	49	6	454
Elbow Macaroni, Deli Salad	1 salad (5 oz)	23	21	2	275
Fresh Fruit, Deli Salad, Small	1 salad	21	18	3	86
Fresh Fruit, Deli Salad	1 salad	30	25	5	123
Homestyle Coleslaw	1 serving (5 oz)	24	21	3	188
Mustard Potato Salad	1 serving (5 oz)	31	27	4	250
Potato Salad	1 serving (5 oz)	35	29	4	288
SUBWAY					
Garden Fresh	1 salad	11	6	5	60
Mediterranean Chicken	1 salad	11	6	5	170
Grilled Chicken & Spinach	1 salad	10	5	5	420
Classic Club	1 salad	14	9	4	390
T.G.I. FRIDAY'S					
Grilled Chicken Caesar Salad	1 serving	na	9	na	na
WENDY'S					
Caesar Side Salad	1 serving	2	1	1	70
Chicken BLT Salad	1 serving	10	6	4	360
Homestyle Chicken Strips Salad	1 serving	34	29	5	450
Mandarin Chicken Salad	1 serving	17	14	3	190
Side Salad	1 serving	7	4	3	35

FAST FOOD AND OTHER RESTAURANTS

FOOD	SERVING	TOTAL CARBS (G)	NET CARBS (G)	FIBER (G)	CALORIES
Spring Mix Salad	1 serving	12	7	5	180
Taco Supreme Salad	1 serving	29	21	8	360

SANDWICHES

ARBY'S

Roast Beef Sandwiches

FOOD	SERVING	TOTAL CARBS (G)	NET CARBS (G)	FIBER (G)	CALORIES
Arby's Melt w/Cheddar	1 sandwich	36	34	2	340
Arby-Q	1 sandwich	40	38	2	360
Beef 'n Cheddar	1 sandwich	43	41	2	480
Big Montana	1 sandwich	41	38	3	630
Giant Roast Beef	1 sandwich	41	38	3	480
Junior Roast Beef	1 sandwich	34	32	2	310
Regular Roast Beef	1 sandwich	34	32	2	350
Super Roast Beef	1 sandwich	47	44	3	470

Other Sandwiches

FOOD	SERVING	TOTAL CARBS (G)	NET CARBS (G)	FIBER (G)	CALORIES
Chicken Bacon 'n Swiss	1 sandwich	49	47	2	610
Chicken Breast Fillet	1 sandwich	47	45	2	540
Chicken Cordon Bleu	1 sandwich	47	45	2	630
Grilled Chicken Deluxe	1 sandwich	39	37	2	410
Roast Chicken Deluxe	1 sandwich	38	36	2	520
Hot Ham 'n Cheese	1 sandwich	35	34	1	340

Market Fresh Sandwiches

FOOD	SERVING	TOTAL CARBS (G)	NET CARBS (G)	FIBER (G)	CALORIES
Roast Beef & Swiss	1 sandwich	73	68	5	810
Roast Ham & Swiss	1 sandwich	74	69	5	730
Roast Chicken Caesar	1 sandwich	75	70	5	820
Roast Turkey & Swiss	1 sandwich	75	70	5	760
Roast Turkey Ranch & Bacon	1 sandwich	74	69	5	880
Market Fresh Ultimate BLT	1 sandwich	72	67	5	820

FAST FOOD AND OTHER RESTAURANTS 175

FOOD	SERVING	TOTAL CARBS (G)	NET CARBS (G)	FIBER (G)	CALORIES
LTO Items (Limited Time Only)					
These items may be available only at participating Arby's franchises.					
Italian Beef 'n Provolone	1 sandwich	54	51	3	650
Philly Beef Supreme	1 sandwich	56	53	3	730
Arby's Low Carbys LTO Items (Limited Time Only)					
These items may be available only at participating Arby's franchises.					
Market Fresh Low Carbys Roast Ham & Swiss	1 sandwich	5	5	t	200
Market Fresh Low Carbys Roast Turkey & Swiss	1 sandwich	4	4	t	210
Market Fresh Low Carbys Roast Beef & Swiss	1 sandwich	3	2	1	280
Market Fresh Low Carbys Roast Turkey Ranch & Bacon	1 sandwich	5	5	t	290
Market Fresh Low Carbys Ultimate BLT	1 sandwich	6	5	1	210
Low Carbys Regular Roast Beef	1 sandwich	1	1	t	150
Low Carbys Giant Roast Beef	1 sandwich	1	1	t	240
Low Carbys Big Montana	1 sandwich	1	0	1	380
Low Carbys Beef n' Cheddar	1 sandwich	1	1	t	250
Low Carbys Super Roast Beef	1 sandwich	2	1	1	150

FAST FOOD AND OTHER RESTAURANTS

FOOD	SERVING	TOTAL CARBS (G)	NET CARBS (G)	FIBER (G)	CALORIES
Low Carbys French Dip n' Swiss	1 sandwich	1	1	t	270
Low Carbys Chicken Breast Fillet	1 sandwich	15	15	t	240
Low Carbys Chicken Bacon n' Swiss	1 sandwich	16	16	t	340
Optional Mayonnaise	1 pkt	0	0	0	100
Optional Spicy Brown Honey Mustard	1 pkt	2	2	0	40
Optional Creamy Ranch Spread	1 pkt	1	1	0	170
Optional Arby's Sauce	1 pkt	4	4	0	15
Optional Arby's Horsey Sauce	1 pkt	3	3	0	60
Optional Red Ranch Dressing	1 pkt	5	5	0	70
Optional au Jus	1 pkt	5	5	0	50
Optional Honey Mustard Sauce	1 pkt	4	4	0	100
Optional Cheddar Cheese Sauce	1 pkt	2	2	0	30
BURGER KING					
Original WHOPPER Sandwich	1 sandwich (291 g)	52	48	4	700
Original WHOPPER Sandwich w/o Mayo	1 sandwich (270 g)	52	48	4	540
Original WHOPPER Sandwich, Low Carb	1 sandwich (167 g)	3	3	t	280
Original WHOPPER Sandwich w/Cheese	1 sandwich (316 g)	53	49	4	800

FAST FOOD AND OTHER RESTAURANTS

FOOD	SERVING	TOTAL CARBS (G)	NET CARBS (G)	FIBER (G)	CALORIES
Original WHOPPER w/Cheese w/o Mayo	1 sandwich (294 g)	53	49	4	640
Original WHOPPER Sandwich w/ Cheese, Low Carb	1 sandwich (192 g)	5	5	t	370
Original Double WHOPPER Sandwich	1 sandwich (374 g)	52	48	4	970
Original Double WHOPPER Sandwich w/o Mayo	1 sandwich (353 g)	52	48	4	810
Original Double WHOPPER Sandwich, Low Carb	1 sandwich (251 g)	3	3	t	540
Original WHOPPER JR. Sandwich	1 sandwich (158 g)	31	29	2	390
Original WHOPPER JR. Sandwich w/o Mayo	1 sandwich (147 g)	31	29	2	310
Original WHOPPER JR. Sandwich, Low Carb	1 sandwich (75 g)	1	1	0	140
Original WHOPPER JR. Sandwich w/Cheese	1 sandwich (160 g)	32	30	2	430
Original WHOPPER JR. Sandwich w/Cheese w/o Mayo	1 sandwich (149 g)	32	30	2	350
Original WHOPPER JR. Sandwich w/ Cheese, Low Carb	1 sandwich (87 g)	2	2	0	190
ADD: Bacon	3 strips	0	0	0	25
Fire-Grilled Hamburger	1 sandwich (121 g)	30	29	1	310
Fire-Grilled Cheeseburger	1 sandwich (133 g)	31	30	1	350

FAST FOOD AND OTHER RESTAURANTS

FOOD	SERVING	TOTAL CARBS (G)	NET CARBS (G)	FIBER (G)	CALORIES
Fire-Grilled Double Hamburger	1 sandwich (164 g)	30	29	1	440
Fire-Grilled Double Cheeseburger	1 sandwich (189 g)	32	30	2	530
Fire-Grilled Bacon Cheeseburger	1 sandwich (141 g)	31	30	1	390
Fire-Grilled Bacon Double Cheeseburger	1 sandwich (196 g)	32	30	2	570
Fire-Grilled, The Angus Steak Burger	1 sandwich (282 g)	62	59	3	640
Fire-Grilled, The Angus Steak Burger, Low Carb	1 sandwich (174 g)	5	5	t	174
Fire-Grilled, The Angus Bacon & Cheese	1 sandwich (317 g)	64	61	3	790
Fire-Grilled, The Angus Bacon & Cheese, Low Carb	1 sandwich (209 g)	7	6	1	500
BK Veggie Burger	1 sandwich (186 g)	46	42	4	380
BK Veggie Burger w/o Mayo	1 sandwich (176 g)	46	42	4	300
Chicken WHOPPER Sandwich	1 sandwich (272 g)	48	44	4	570
Chicken WHOPPER Sandwich w/o Mayo	1 sandwich (251 g)	48	44	4	410
Chicken WHOPPER Sandwich, Low Carb	1 sandwich (163 g)	3	2	1	160
Original Chicken Sandwich	1 sandwich (204 g)	52	49	3	560
Original Chicken Sandwich w/o Mayo	1 sandwich (190 g)	52	49	3	460

FAST FOOD AND OTHER RESTAURANTS 179

FOOD	SERVING	TOTAL CARBS (G)	NET CARBS (G)	FIBER (G)	CALORIES
TenderCrisp Chicken Sandwich	1 sandwich (310 g)	72	66	6	810
TenderCrisp Chicken Sandwich w/o Mayo	1 sandwich (281 g)	71	65	6	600
Spicy TenderCrisp Chicken Sandwich	1 sandwich (310 g)	73	67	6	750
CHICKEN TENDERS	4 pieces	10	10	0	170
CHICKEN TENDERS	5 pieces	13	13	t	210
CHICKEN TENDERS	6 pieces	15	15	t	250
CHICKEN TENDERS	8 pieces	20	20	t	340
BK FISH FILET Sandwich	1 sandwich (185 g)	44	42	2	520
BK FISH FILET Sandwich w/o Tartar Sauce	1 sandwich (156 g)	42	40	2	360 |//
CHICK-FIL-A:					
Chick-fil-A Chicken Sandwich	1 sandwich (6 g)	38	37	1	410
Chick-fil-A Chicken Sandwich w/o Butter	1 sandwich (5.8 g)	37	36	1	380
Chicken Deluxe Sandwich	1 sandwich (7.3 g)	39	37	2	420
Chicken, Filet Only, No Bun, No Pickles	1 filet (3.7 g)	10	10	0	230
Chick-fil-A Chargrilled Chicken Sandwich	1 sandwich (5.53 g)	30	29	280	250
Chick-fil-A Chargrilled Chicken Sandwich, w/o Butter	1 sandwich (5.33 g)	28	27	1	250

FAST FOOD AND OTHER RESTAURANTS

FOOD	SERVING	TOTAL CARBS (G)	NET CARBS (G)	FIBER (G)	CALORIES
Chick-fil-A Chargrilled Chicken Deluxe Sandwich	1 sandwich (6.87 g)	31	29	2	250
Chick-fil-A Chargrilled Chicken Deluxe Sandwich, w/o Butter	1 sandwich (6.67 g)	31	29	2	290
Chargrilled Chicken, Filet Only, No Bun, No Pickles	1 filet (3.2 g)	1	1	0	100
Chargrilled Chicken Club Sandwich, No Sauce	1 sandwich (7.57 g)	31	29	2	370
Chick-fil-A Chicken Salad Sandwich, on Wheat Bread	1 sandwich (5.4 g)	32	27	5	350
CHILI'S					
Bunless Style Burger, Low Carb, Bacon Burger w/ Cheese & Mayo & Side of Veggies (No Bun, No Fries)	1 order	9	3	6	640
Bunless Style Burger, Low Carb, Mushroom Swiss w/Mayo & Side of Veggies (No Bun, No Fries)	1 order	14	8	6	602
Bunless Style Burger, Low Carb, Old Timer w/Mustard & Side of Veggies (No Bun, No Fries)	1 order	11	5	6	574

FAST FOOD AND OTHER RESTAURANTS

FOOD	SERVING	TOTAL CARBS (G)	NET CARBS (G)	FIBER (G)	CALORIES
Guiltless Grill Chicken Pita, w/Low Fat Ranch Dressing & Black Beans	1 order	77	62	15	545
Guiltless Grill Chicken Sandwich, w/Low Fat Honey Mustard & Steamed Fresh Veggies & Black Beans	1 order	70	59	11	527
DAIRY QUEEN					
BBQ Beef Sandwich	1 serving	37	35	2	300
BBQ Pork Sandwich	1 serving	36	34	2	280
Breaded Chicken Sandwich	1 serving	47	43	4	510
Grilled Chicken Sandwich	1 serving	30	27	3	310
Hot Dog	1 serving	19	18	1	240
Chili n' Cheese Dog	1 serving	22	20	2	330
Super Dog	1 serving	39	37	2	580
Super Dog Chili n' Cheese	1 serving	42	39	3	710
DENNY'S					
Carb Watch Burger	1 sandwich	13	10	3	625
Club Sandwich	1 sandwich	45	43	2	602
The Super Bird Sandwich	1 sandwich	32	30	2	479
Grilled Chicken Sandwich w/o Dressing	1 sandwich	56	52	4	476
Bacon, Lettuce & Tomato	1 sandwich	50	48	2	610
BBQ Chicken Sandwich	1 sandwich	86	81	5	1,089
Classic Burger	1 sandwich	56	52	4	694
Classic Burger w/Cheese	1 sandwich	57	53	4	852

182 FAST FOOD AND OTHER RESTAURANTS

FOOD	SERVING	TOTAL CARBS (G)	NET CARBS (G)	FIBER (G)	CALORIES
Hickory Cheeseburger	1 sandwich	84	79	5	1,221
Bacon Cheddar Burger	1 sandwich	58	53	5	875
Patty Melt	1 sandwich	37	43	4	798
Chicken Ranch Melt	1 sandwich	44	41	3	758
Hoagie Chicken Melt	1 sandwich	43	42	2	751
Hoagie Philly Melt	1 sandwich	58	53	5	874
Boca Burger	1 sandwich	64	55	9	601
Mushroom Swiss Burger	1 sandwich	63	58	5	880
Buffalo Chicken Sandwich	1 sandwich	80	75	5	708
Turkey Breast on Multigrain w/o Mayo	1 sandwich	41	36	5	277
Ham & Swiss on Rye w/o Mayo	1 sandwich	39	34	5	417
Albacore Tuna Melt	1 sandwich	42	39	3	640
HARDEE'S					
⅓ lb Thickburger	1 sandwich	54	51	3	850
⅓ lb Cheeseburger	1 sandwich	51	48	3	680
⅓ lb Mushroom N Swiss Thickburger	1 sandwich	48	46	2	720
⅓ lb Bacon Cheese Thickburger	1 sandwich	50	47	3	910
⅓ lb Chili Cheese Thickburger	1 sandwich	55	51	4	870
⅓ lb Low Carb Thickburger	1 sandwich	5	3	2	420
½ lb Six Dollar Burger	1 sandwich	72	67	5	1,120
½ lb Grilled Sourdough Thickburger	1 sandwich	61	56	5	1,100

FOOD	SERVING	TOTAL CARBS (G)	NET CARBS (G)	FIBER (G)	CALORIES
⅔ lb Bacon Cheese Thickburger	1 sandwich	60	55	5	1,340
⅔ lb Double Thickburger	1 sandwich	53	50	3	1,230
⅔ lb Double Bacon Cheese Thickburger	1 sandwich	51	48	3	1,300
Charbroiled Chicken Sandwich	1 sandwich	53	49	4	590
Low Carb Charbroiled Chicken Sandwich	1 sandwich	11	9	2	420
Big Chicken Sandwich	1 sandwich	73	69	4	770
Spicy Chicken Sandwich	1 sandwich	46	44	2	430
Regular Roast Beef	1 sandwich	29	27	2	330
Big Roast Beef	1 sandwich	38	36	2	470
Hot Ham 'n Cheese	1 sandwich	39	37	2	420
Big Hot Ham 'n Cheese	1 sandwich	59	56	3	570
Hot Dog	1 sandwich	22	21	1	420
Slammer	1 sandwich	19	19	0	240
Slammer w/Cheese	1 sandwich	20	20	0	140
Kids Meal, Slammers	1 meal	71	67	4	720
JACK IN THE BOX					
Deli Trio Pannido	1 sandwich	53	51	2	645
Ham & Turkey Pannido	1 sandwich	54	52	2	610
Zesty Turkey Pannido	1 sandwich	51	49	2	740
Ultimate Club Sandwich	1 sandwich	52	50	2	630
Chicken Fajita Pita	1 pita	33	33	0	315
Chicken Sandwich	1 sandwich	39	38	1	390
Chicken Sandwich w/Cheese	1 sandwich	40	39	1	430
Jack's Spicy Chicken	1 sandwich	62	59	3	615

FAST FOOD AND OTHER RESTAURANTS

FOOD	SERVING	TOTAL CARBS (G)	NET CARBS (G)	FIBER (G)	CALORIES
Jack's Spicy Chicken w/Cheese	1 sandwich	63	60	3	695
Sourdough Grilled Chicken Club	1 sandwich	35	33	2	505
Southwest Pita	1 pita	35	31	4	260
Bacon Bacon Cheeseburger	1 sandwich	50	48	2	780
Bacon Ultimate Cheeseburger	1 sandwich	53	51	2	1,025
Hamburger	1 sandwich	30	30	0	310
Hamburger w/Cheese	1 sandwich	31	31	0	355
Hamburger Deluxe	1 sandwich	32	32	0	370
Hamburger Deluxe w/Cheese	1 sandwich	34	34	0	460
Jumbo Jack	1 sandwich	52	50	2	600
Jumbo Jack w/Cheese	1 sandwich	55	54	2	695
Junior Bacon Cheeseburger	1 sandwich	32	32	0	525
Sourdough Jack	1 sandwich	36	34	2	715
Ultimate Cheeseburger	1 sandwich	52	50	2	945
KFC (KENTUCKY FRIED CHICKEN)					
Original Recipe Sandwich w/Sauce	1 sandwich	22	22	0	450
Original Recipe Sandwich w/o Sauce	1 sandwich	21	21	0	320
TC Sandwich w/Sauce	1 sandwich	42	41	1	670
TC Sandwich w/o Sauce	1 sandwich	41	40	1	540
Zinger Sandwich w/Sauce	1 sandwich	42	41	1	680

FOOD	SERVING	TOTAL CARBS (G)	NET CARBS (G)	FIBER (G)	CALORIES
Zinger Sandwich w/o Sauce	1 sandwich	41	40	1	540
TR Sandwich w/Sauce	1 sandwich	24	23	1	390
TR Sandwich w/o Sauce	1 sandwich	23	22	1	260
Hot BBQ Sandwich	1 sandwich	41	37	4	300
Twister	1 sandwich	55	52	3	670
LONG JOHN SILVER'S					
Fish Sandwich	1 sandwich	48	45	3	440
Ultimate Fish Sandwich	1 sandwich	48	45	3	500
Chicken Sandwich	1 sandwich	41	38	3	360
MCDONALD'S					
Hamburger	1 sandwich	36	34	2	280
Cheeseburger	1 sandwich	36	34	2	330
Double Cheeseburger	1 sandwich	38	36	2	490
Quarter Pounder	1 sandwich	38	35	3	430
Quarter Pounder w/Cheese	1 sandwich	39	36	3	540
Double Quarter Pounder w/Cheese	1 sandwich	39	36	3	770
Big Mac	1 sandwich	50	46	4	600
Big N' Tasty w/Cheese	1 sandwich	39	36	3	590
Filet-O-Fish	1 sandwich	41	40	1	410
Chicken McGrill	1 sandwich	37	34	3	400
Crispy Chicken	1 sandwich	47	44	3	510
McChicken	1 sandwich	41	38	3	430
Hot 'n Spicy McChicken	1 sandwich	40	39	1	450
RUBY TUESDAY					
Alpine Burger	1 sandwich	na	53	5	1,081
American Cheeseburger	1 sandwich	na	49	3	942

FAST FOOD AND OTHER RESTAURANTS

FOOD	SERVING	TOTAL CARBS (G)	NET CARBS (G)	FIBER (G)	CALORIES
Bacon Cheeseburger	1 sandwich	na	49	3	1,009
Black & Bleu Burger	1 sandwich	na	53	3	995
Classic Burger	1 sandwich	na	48	3	830
Colossal Burger	1 sandwich	na	73	5	1,677
Old English Bacon Cheeseburger	1 sandwich	na	49	3	1,076
Pepper Jack Bacon Burger	1 sandwich	na	53	3	1,134
Smokehouse Burger	1 sandwich	na	70	4	1,144
Thai-One-On Burger	1 sandwich	na	57	3	1,119
Veggie Burger	1 sandwich	na	67	5	610
Buffalo & Bleu Sandwich	1 sandwich	na	64	3	1,020
Crispy Chicken Club	1 sandwich	na	60	3	830
Hickory Chicken Sandwich	1 sandwich	na	62	3	854
Roasted Turkey BLT	1 sandwich	na	67	5	1,149
The Killer Fish Sandwich	1 sandwich	na	48	3	920
The Ultimate Roasted Turkey Sandwich	1 sandwich	na	66	5	919
SCHLOTZSKY'S DELI					
The Original on Sourdough Bun, Small	1 sandwich	53	50	3	525
The Original on Sourdough Bun, Regular	1 sandwich	79	75	4	738
Large Original on Sourdough Bun, Family Size	1 sandwich	152	145	7	1,390

FOOD	SERVING	TOTAL CARBS (G)	NET CARBS (G)	FIBER (G)	CALORIES
Deluxe Original on Sourdough Bun, Small	1 sandwich	57	54	3	693
Deluxe Original on Sourdough Bun, Regular	1 sandwich	84	80	4	930
Ham & Cheese on Sourdough Bun, Small	1 sandwich	55	52	3	512
Ham & Cheese on Sourdough Bun, Regular	1 sandwich	82	78	4	749
Turkey Original on Sourdough Bun, Small	1 sandwich	54	51	3	583
Turkey Original on Sourdough Bun, Regular	1 sandwich	81	77	4	822
Albacore Tuna on Wheat Bun, Small	1 sandwich	52	49	3	334
Albacore Tuna on Wheat Bun, Regular	1 sandwich	77	72	5	496
Albacore Tuna Melt on Wheat Bun, Small	1 sandwich	56	52	4	509
Albacore Tuna Melt on Wheat Bun, Regular	1 sandwich	83	77	6	740
BLT on Sourdough Bun, Small	1 sandwich	47	45	2	379
BLT on Sourdough Bun, Small	1 sandwich	70	67	3	578

FAST FOOD AND OTHER RESTAURANTS

FOOD	SERVING	TOTAL CARBS (G)	NET CARBS (G)	FIBER (G)	CALORIES
Chicken Breast on Sourdough Bun, Small	1 sandwich	54	51	3	337
Chicken Breast on Sourdough Bun, Regular	1 sandwich	80	76	4	499
Chicken Club on Sourdough Bun, Small	1 sandwich	50	47	3	458
Chicken Club on Sourdough Bun, Regular	1 sandwich	75	71	4	686
Corned Beef on Dark Rye Bun, Small	1 sandwich	52	49	3	393
Corned Beef on Dark Rye Bun, Regular	1 sandwich	78	74	4	593
Corned Beef Reuben on Dark Rye Bun, Small	1 sandwich	55	52	3	534
Corned Beef Reuben on Dark Rye Bun, Regular	1 sandwich	82	78	4	838
Dijon Chicken on Wheat Bun, Small	1 sandwich	49	45	4	329
Dijon Chicken on Wheat Bun, Regular	1 sandwich	74	68	6	496
Fiesta Chicken on Jalapeño Cheese Bun, Small	1 sandwich	53	50	3	577

FOOD	SERVING	TOTAL CARBS (G)	NET CARBS (G)	FIBER (G)	CALORIES
Fiesta Chicken on Jalapeño Cheese Bun, Regular	1 sandwich	79	75	4	839
Pastrami & Swiss on Dark Rye Bun, Small	1 sandwich	54	51	3	586
Pastrami & Swiss on Dark Rye Bun, Regular	1 sandwich	81	77	4	882
Pastrami Reuben on Dark Rye Bun, Small	1 sandwich	56	53	3	635
Pastrami Reuben on Dark Rye Bun, Regular	1 sandwich	83	79	4	944
Pesto Chicken on Sourdough Bun, Small	1 sandwich	49	47	2	346
Pesto Chicken on Sourdough Bun, Regular	1 sandwich	73	69	4	512
Roast Beef on Sourdough Bun, Small	1 sandwich	52	50	2	418
Roast Beef on Sourdough Bun, Regular	1 sandwich	78	75	3	623
Roast Beef & Cheese on Sourdough Bun, Small	1 sandwich	56	53	3	586

FAST FOOD AND OTHER RESTAURANTS

FOOD	SERVING	TOTAL CARBS (G)	NET CARBS (G)	FIBER (G)	CALORIES
Roast Beef & Cheese on Sourdough Bun, Regular	1 sandwich	83	79	4	855
Santa Fe Chicken on Jalapeño Cheese Bun, Small	1 sandwich	54	51	3	404
Santa Fe Chicken on Jalapeño Cheese Bun, Regular	1 sandwich	81	76	5	605
Smoked Turkey Breast on Sourdough Bun, Small	1 sandwich	50	48	2	335
Smoked Turkey Breast on Sourdough Bun, Regular	1 sandwich	75	72	3	498
Texas Schlotzsky's on Jalapeño Cheese Bun, Small	1 sandwich	51	49	2	537
Texas Schlotzsky's on Jalapeño Cheese Bun, Regular	1 sandwich	76	73	3	776
The Philly on Sourdough Bun, Small	1 sandwich	57	55	2	571
The Philly on Sourdough Bun, Regular	1 sandwich	86	82	4	840
The Vegetarian on Sourdough Bun, Small	1 sandwich	53	49	4	324

FOOD	SERVING	TOTAL CARBS (G)	NET CARBS (G)	FIBER (G)	CALORIES
The Vegetarian on Sourdough Bun, Regular	1 sandwich	79	73	6	482
Turkey & Bacon Club on Sourdough Bun, Small	1 sandwich	53	50	3	571
Turkey & Bacon Club on Sourdough Bun, Regular	1 sandwich	79	74	5	834
Turkey Guacamole on Sourdough Bun, Small	1 sandwich	56	54	2	423
Turkey Guacamole on Sourdough Bun, Regular	1 sandwich	84	81	3	643
Turkey Reuben on Dark Rye Bun, Small	1 sandwich	54	51	3	554
Turkey Reuben on Dark Rye Bun, Regular	1 sandwich	80	76	4	823
Vegetable Club on Sourdough Bun, Small	1 sandwich	50	47	3	367
Vegetable Club on Sourdough Bun, Regular	1 sandwich	76	71	5	541
Western Vegetarian on Sourdough Bun, Small	1 sandwich	51	49	3	425

FAST FOOD AND OTHER RESTAURANTS

FOOD	SERVING	TOTAL CARBS (G)	NET CARBS (G)	FIBER (G)	CALORIES
Western Vegetarian on Sourdough Bun, Regular	1 sandwich	76	72	4	611
Kids' Cheese Sandwich on Sourdough Bun	1 sandwich	49	46	2	401
Kids' PBJ on Sourdough Bun	1 sandwich	71	67	4	470
Kids' Ham & Cheese Sandwich on Sourdough Bun	1 sandwich	50	48	2	431

SONIC

FOOD	SERVING	TOTAL CARBS (G)	NET CARBS (G)	FIBER (G)	CALORIES
No. 1 Sonic Burger	1 sandwich	43	41	2	577
No. 2 Sonic Burger	1 sandwich	43	41	2	481
No. 1 Sonic Cheeseburger	1 sandwich	44	42	2	647
No. 2 Sonic Cheeseburger	1 sandwich	44	42	2	551
Bacon Cheeseburger	1 sandwich	44	42	2	727
SuperSonic No. 1	1 sandwich	45	43	2	929
SuperSonic No. 2	1 sandwich	46	43	3	839
Jr. Burger	1 sandwich	27	26	1	353
Grilled Cheese Toaster Sandwich	1 sandwich	39	37	2	282
BLT Toaster Sandwich	1 sandwich	42	39	3	581
Bacon Cheddar Burger Toaster Sandwich	1 sandwich	60	56	4	675
Chicken Club Toaster Sandwich	1 sandwich	75	72	3	675
Country Fried Steak Toaster Sandwich	1 sandwich	55	52	3	708

FOOD	SERVING	TOTAL CARBS (G)	NET CARBS (G)	FIBER (G)	CALORIES
Country Fried Steak Sandwich	1 sandwich	56	54	2	748
Grilled Chicken Sandwich	1 sandwich	31	29	2	343
Breaded Chicken Sandwich	1 sandwich	66	64	2	582
Regular Cheese Coney	1 sandwich	24	23	1	366
Regular Coney Plain	1 sandwich	22	21	1	262
Extra Long Cheese Coney	1 sandwich	47	45	2	666
Extra Long Coney Plain	1 sandwich	44	43	1	483
Corn Dog	1 sandwich	23	22	1	262
Hot Dog Plain	1 sandwich	22	21	1	262
WENDY'S					
Jr. Hamburger	1 sandwich	34	32	2	270
Jr. Cheeseburger	1 sandwich	34	32	2	310
Jr. Cheeseburger Deluxe	1 sandwich	36	34	2	350
Jr. Bacon Cheeseburger	1 sandwich	34	32	2	380
Hamburger, Kids' Meal	1 sandwich	33	32	1	270
Cheeseburger, Kids' Meal	1 sandwich	33	32	1	310
Classic Single w/Everything	1 sandwich	37	35	2	410
Big Bacon Classic	1 sandwich	45	42	3	580
Ultimate Chicken Grill Sandwich	1 sandwich	44	42	2	360
Spicy Chicken Fillet Sandwich	1 sandwich	57	55	2	510
Homestyle Chicken Fillet Sandwich	1 sandwich	57	55	2	540

SIDE ITEMS AND OTHER INDIVIDUAL ITEMS

ARBY'S

FOOD	SERVING	TOTAL CARBS (G)	NET CARBS (G)	FIBER (G)	CALORIES
Cheddar Curly Fries	1 serving (6 oz)	54	50	4	460
Curly Fries, Small	1 serving (3.5 oz)	39	36	3	310
Curly Fries, Medium	1 serving (4.5 oz)	50	46	4	400
Curly Fries, Large	1 serving (7 oz)	78	71	7	198
Homestyle Fries, Child-Size	1 serving (3 oz)	32	29	3	220
Homestyle Fries, Small	1 serving (4 oz)	42	39	3	300
Homestyle Fries, Medium	1 serving	53	49	4	370
Homestyle Fries, Large	1 serving	79	73	6	560
Potato Cakes	2 cakes (3.5 oz)	26	23	3	250
Jalapeño Bites	1 serving (4 oz)	30	28	2	330
Mozzarella Sticks	4 sticks (4.8 oz)	34	32	2	470
Onion Petals	1 serving (4 oz)	43	41	3	410
Chicken Finger Snack w/Curly Fries	1 serving (6.4 oz)	55	52	3	580
Chicken Finger 4-Pack	1 serving (6.77 oz)	42	42	0	640
Baked Potato w/Butter & Sour Cream	1 potato (11.2 oz)	65	59	6	500
Broccoli 'N Cheddar Baked Potato	1 potato (14 oz)	71	64	7	540
Deluxe Baked Potato	1 potato (13 oz)	67	61	6	650

BLIMPIE

FOOD	SERVING	TOTAL CARBS (G)	NET CARBS (G)	FIBER (G)	CALORIES
Coleslaw	5 oz	13	12	1	180
Macaroni Salad	5 oz	25	24	1	360
Mustard Potato Salad	5 oz	21	20	1	160
Potato Salad	5 oz	19	18	1	270

FOOD	SERVING	TOTAL CARBS (G)	NET CARBS (G)	FIBER (G)	CALORIES
BURGER KING					
French Fries, Small	1 serving	29	27	2	100
French Fries, Medium	1 serving	46	42	4	360
French Fries, Large	1 serving	63	58	5	500
French Fries, King	1 serving	76	70	6	600
Onion Rings, Small	1 serving	22	20	2	180
Onion Rings, Medium	1 serving	40	37	3	320
Onion Rings, Large	1 serving	60	55	5	480
Onion Rings, King	1 serving	70	65	5	550
Chili	1 serving	17	12	5	190
ADD: Cheddar Cheese Shredded	1 serving	0	0	0	90
ADD: Crackers	1 serving	4	4	0	25
CHICK-FIL-A					
Chick-fil-A Chick-N-Strips	4 strips (4.48 g)	14	13	1	290
Chick-fil-A Nuggets	8 nuggets (4 g)	12	12	t	260
Side Salad	1 salad (3.8 g)	4	2	2	60
Coleslaw	1 small (3.7 g)	14	12	2	210
Carrot & Raisin Salad	1 small (3.2 g)	22	20	2	130
Chick-fil-A Waffle Potato Fries	1 small (3 g)	37	32	5	280
CHILI'S					
Buffalo Wings Starter, Low Carb w/Celery & Blue Cheese Dressing	1 order	5	2	3	790
DAIRY QUEEN					
French Fries, Small	1 small order	45	42	3	300

FAST FOOD AND OTHER RESTAURANTS

FOOD	SERVING	TOTAL CARBS (G)	NET CARBS (G)	FIBER (G)	CALORIES
French Fries, Medium	1 medium order	56	52	4	380
French Fries, Large	1 large order	72	67	5	480
Onion Rings	1 order	45	42	3	470
DENNY'S					
Corn in Butter Sauce	1 serving	18	17	1	93
Carrots in Sauce	1 serving	8	6	2	50
Green Beans in Sauce	1 serving	5	3	2	40
Baked Potato, Plain w/Skin	1 serving	51	46	5	220
Mashed Potatoes, Plain	1 serving	23	21	2	168
Bread Stuffing, Plain	1 serving	19	18	1	100
Cottage Cheese	1 serving	2	2	0	72
Apple Sauce, Musselman's	1 serving	15	14	1	60
Sliced Tomatoes	3 slices	3	2	1	13
French Fries	1 serving	57	52	5	423
Seasoned Fries	1 serving	35	35	0	261
Onion Rings	1 serving	38	37	1	381
DOMINO'S					
Breadsticks w/o Sauce	1 stick	12	12	0	115
Cheesy Bread w/o Sauce	1 stick	13	13	0	123
Marinara Dipping Sauce	1 container	5	5	0	25
Garlic Sauce	1 container	0	0	0	440
Cinna Stix	1 stick	15	14	1	123
Sweet Icing	1 container	57	57	0	250
Domino's Pizza Buffalo Chicken Kickers w/o Sauce	1 piece	3	3	0	47
Hot Buffalo Wings	1 wing	1	1	0	45

FAST FOOD AND OTHER RESTAURANTS 197

FOOD	SERVING	TOTAL CARBS (G)	NET CARBS (G)	FIBER (G)	CALORIES
Barbecue Buffalo Wings	1 wing	2	2	0	50
Hot Dipping Sauce	1 container	4	4	0	15
Blue Cheese Dipping Sauce	1 container	2	2	0	223
Ranch Dipping Sauce	1 container	2	2	0	197
HARDEE'S					
Cinnamon Roll	1 roll	96	94	2	390
Grits	1 serving	16	16	0	110
Hash Rounds, Small	1 small serving	25	23	2	260
Hash Rounds, Medium	1 medium serving	34	31	3	350
Hash Rounds, Large	1 large serving	45	41	4	460
Croissant	1 croissant	26	26	0	210
JACK IN THE BOX					
Bacon Cheddar Potato Wedges	1 serving	45	40	5	620
Egg Roll	1 roll	26	24	2	175
Egg Rolls	3 rolls	55	49	6	445
Stuffed Jalapeños	3 pieces	22	20	2	230
Stuffed Jalapeños	7 pieces	51	47	4	530
French Fries, Small	1 serving	44	41	3	330
French Fries, Medium	1 serving	55	51	4	410
French Fries, Large	1 serving	77	71	6	580
Onion Rings	1 serving	51	48	3	500
Seasoned Curly Fries, Small	1 serving	30	27	3	270
Seasoned Curly Fries, Medium	1 serving	45	40	5	400
Seasoned Curly Fries, Large	1 serving	60	54	6	550

FAST FOOD AND OTHER RESTAURANTS

FOOD	SERVING	TOTAL CARBS (G)	NET CARBS (G)	FIBER (G)	CALORIES
KFC (KENTUCKY FRIED CHICKEN)					
Biscuit	1 biscuit	23	23	0	190
Green Beans	1 serving	5	3	2	50
Mashed Potatoes w/o Gravy	1 serving	16	15	1	110
Mashed Potatoes w/Gravy	1 serving	18	17	1	120
Macaroni & Cheese	1 serving	15	14	1	130
Potato Wedges, Small Size	1 serving	30	27	3	240
Corn on the Cob	1 cob, 3" large	13	10	3	70
Corn on the Cob	1 cob, 5.5" large	26	19	7	150
BBQ Beans	1 serving	46	39	7	230
Potato Salad	1 serving	22	21	1	180
Coleslaw	1 serving	22	19	3	190
LONG JOHN SILVER'S					
Regular Fries	1 serving	34	31	3	230
Large Fries	1 serving	56	51	5	390
Hushpuppies	1 pup	9	6	3	60
Slaw	1 serving	15	12	3	200
Corn Cobbette	1 cobbette	14	11	3	90
Cheese Sticks	3 sticks	12	11	1	140
Rice	1 serving	34	31	3	180
Crumblies	1 serving	14	13	1	170
Clam Chowder	1 bowl	23	23	t	220
MCDONALD'S					
Small French Fries	1 serving	28	25	3	220
Medium French Fries	1 serving	44	40	4	350
Large French Fries	1 serving	66	60	6	520

FAST FOOD AND OTHER RESTAURANTS

FOOD	SERVING	TOTAL CARBS (G)	NET CARBS (G)	FIBER (G)	CALORIES
PAPA JOHN'S					
Cheese Sticks	1 serving	20	19	1	68
Bread Sticks	1 serving	26	25	1	55
Papa's ChickenStrips	1 serving	5	5	t	37
Cheese Sauce	1 serving	0	0	0	35
Garlic Sauce	1 serving	0	0	0	35
Pizza Sauce	1 serving	3	1	2	35
PIZZA HUT					
Hot Wings	2 wings	1	1	0	110
Mild Wings	2 wings	t	t	0	110
Wing Ranch Dipping Sauce	1 serving (1.5 oz)	4	4	0	210
Wing Blue Cheese Dipping Sauce	1 serving (1.5 oz)	2	2	0	230
Breadsticks	1 breadstick	20	20	t	150
Cheese Breadsticks	1 breadstick	21	21	t	200
RUBY TUESDAY					
Creamed Spinach, Low Carb	1 serving	na	9	2	204
Fresh Steamed Broccoli, Low Carb	1 serving	na	1	4	38
Sugar Snap Peas, Low Carb	1 serving	na	10	4	82
Creamy Mashed Cauliflower, Low Carb	1 serving	na	9	6	166
Fresh Sautéed Zucchini	1 serving	na	3	2	54
Baked Potato	1 serving	na	62	14	375
Mashed Potatoes	1 serving	na	29	6	265

FAST FOOD AND OTHER RESTAURANTS

FOOD	SERVING	TOTAL CARBS (G)	NET CARBS (G)	FIBER (G)	CALORIES
Ruby's Fries	1 serving	na	19	5	185
Brown Rice Pilaf	1 serving	na	33	2	194
Onion Straw	1 serving	na	31	3	426
Coleslaw	1 serving	na	16	0	159
Garlic Toast	1 serving	na	23	1	220
Crackers	2 crackers	na	4	0	26
SONIC					
Regular French Fries	1 serving	22	18	4	195
Regular Cheese Fries	1 serving	23	19	4	265
Regular Chili Cheese Fries	1 serving	24	20	4	299
Large French Fries	1 serving	30	25	5	252
Large Cheese Fries	1 serving	31	26	5	322
Large Chili Cheese Fries	1 serving	32	27	5	357
SuperSonic Fries	1 serving	44	37	7	358
Regular Tater Tots	1 serving	27	25	3	259
Regular Cheese Tater Tots	1 serving	28	25	3	329
Regular Chili Cheese Tater Tots	1 serving	28	25	3	363
Large Tater Tots	1 serving	40	36	4	365
Large Cheese Tater Tots	1 serving	41	37	4	435
Large Chili Cheese Tater Tots	1 serving	43	38	5	547
SuperSonic Tots	1 serving	53	48	5	485
Regular Onion Rings	1 serving	66	59	7	331
Large Onion Rings	1 serving	102	92	10	507

FOOD	SERVING	TOTAL CARBS (G)	NET CARBS (G)	FIBER (G)	CALORIES
Sonic Onion Rings	1 serving	141	130	11	706
Fritos Chili Pie	1 serving	36	33	3	611
Mozzarella Sticks	1 serving	35	35	0	382
Ched 'R' Peppers	1 serving	29	25	4	256
Chicken Strips	2 strips	15	15	0	184
SCHLOTZSKY'S DELI					
Barbecue Deli Chips	1 bag (1.5 oz)	26	24	2	210
Cracked Pepper Deli Chips	1 bag (1.5 oz)	25	24	1	210
Jalapeño Deli Chips	1 bag (1.5 oz)	26	24	2	210
Regular (Plain) Deli Chips	1 bag (1.5 oz)	26	24	2	210
Salt & Vinegar Deli Chips	1 bag (1.5 oz)	26	24	2	210
Sour Cream & Onion Deli Chips	1 bag (1.5 oz)	26	24	2	210
WENDY'S					
Baked Potato, Plain	1 potato	61	54	7	270
Baked Potato, Sour Cream & Chives	1 potato	62	55	7	340
Baked Potato, Broccoli & Cheese	1 potato	70	61	9	440
Baked Potato, Bacon & Cheese	1 potato	67	60	7	560
Chili, Small	8 oz	21	16	5	200
Chili, Large	12 oz	31	24	7	300
Hot Chili Seasoning	1 pkt	2	2	0	5
Saltine Crackers	2 crackers	5	5	0	25

FAST FOOD AND OTHER RESTAURANTS

FOOD	SERVING	TOTAL CARBS (G)	NET CARBS (G)	FIBER (G)	CALORIES
Cheddar Cheese, Shredded	2 tbsp	1	1	0	70
French Fries, Kid's Meal	3.2 oz	36	32	4	250
French Fries, Medium	5 oz	56	50	6	390
French Fries, Biggie	5.6 oz	63	56	7	440
French Fries, Great Biggie	6.7 oz	75	67	8	530

SOUPS

BLIMPIE

FOOD	SERVING	TOTAL CARBS (G)	NET CARBS (G)	FIBER (G)	CALORIES
Chicken Soup w/ White & Wild Rice	8 oz	21	19	2	230
Grande Chili w/Beans & Beef	8 oz	30	12	18	250
Vegetable Beef	8 oz	13	11	2	80
Cream of Potato	8 oz	24	21	3	190
Homestyle Chicken Noodle	8 oz	18	17	1	120
Cream of Broccoli & Cheese	8 oz	15	12	3	190
Garden Vegetable	8 oz	14	11	3	80

CHILI'S

FOOD	SERVING	TOTAL CARBS (G)	NET CARBS (G)	FIBER (G)	CALORIES
Beef Chili, Low Carb, w/Cheese, Sour Cream & Pico de Gallo, w/o Crackers	1 order	25	19	6	579
Broccoli Cheese Soup, Low Carb, w/Pico de Gallo, w/o Crackers	1 order	20	18	2	315

FOOD	SERVING	TOTAL CARBS (G)	NET CARBS (G)	FIBER (G)	CALORIES
CHICK-FIL-A					
Hearty Breast of Chicken Soup	1 cup	18	17	1	140
DENNY'S					
Vegetable Beef	1 serving	11	9	2	79
Chicken Noodle	1 serving	8	8	0	60
Cream of Broccoli	1 serving	41	39	2	574
Clam Chowder	1 serving	55	51	4	624
RUBY TUESDAY					
Baked French Onion Soup	1 serving	na	29	1	547
Broccoli & Cheese Soups, Low Carb	1 serving	na	12	3	332
Onion Soup	1 serving	na	20	0	198
White Chicken Chili	1 serving	na	22	6	218
SCHLOTZSKY'S DELI					
Boston Clam Chowder	1 cup (8 oz)	24	23	1	233
Broccoli Cheese w/Florets	1 cup (8 oz)	23	22	1	252
Chicken Gumbo	1 cup (8 oz)	13	11	2	110
Chicken Tortilla	1 cup (8 oz)	13	12	1	150
Chicken w/Wild Rice	1 cup (8 oz)	36	36	0	360
Gourmet Vegetable Beef	1 cup (8 oz)	14	12	2	120
Minestrone	1 cup (8 oz)	17	14	3	89
Monterey Black Bean	1 cup (8 oz)	42	25	17	240
Old-Fashioned Chicken Noodle	1 cup (8 oz)	18	17	1	122
Pilgrim Corn Chowder	1 cup (8 oz)	38	37	1	284
Potato w/Bacon	1 cup (8 oz)	31	29	2	226

FAST FOOD AND OTHER RESTAURANTS

FOOD	SERVING	TOTAL CARBS (G)	NET CARBS (G)	FIBER (G)	CALORIES
Ravioli	1 cup (8 oz)	21	20	1	111
Red Beans & Rice	1 cup (8 oz)	32	28	4	167
Timberline Chili	1 cup (8 oz)	24	17	7	210
Tuscan Tomato Basil	1 cup (8 oz)	13	10	3	320
Vegetarian Vegetable	1 cup (8 oz)	20	14	6	138
Wisconsin Cheese	1 cup (8 oz)	26	25	1	319
SUBWAY					
Brown & Wild Rice w/Chicken	1 cup	17	15	2	190
Chicken & Dumpling	1 cup	16	15	1	130
Chili con Carne	1 cup	23	17	8	240
Cream of Broccoli	1 cup	15	13	2	130
Cream of Potato w/Bacon	1 cup	21	19	2	200
Cream of Ham & Bacon	1 cup	17	16	1	240
Golden Broccoli & Cheese	1 cup	16	14	2	180
Minestrone	1 cup	11	9	2	70
New England Clam Chowder	1 cup	16	15	1	110
Roasted Chicken Noodle	1 cup	7	6	1	60
Spanish Style Chicken w/Rice	1 cup	13	12	1	90
Tomato Garden Vegetable w/Rotini	1 cup	20	18	2	100
Vegetable Beef	1 cup	15	12	3	90

FAST FOOD AND OTHER RESTAURANTS

FOOD	SERVING	TOTAL CARBS (G)	NET CARBS (G)	FIBER (G)	CALORIES
WENDY'S					
Chili, Small	8 oz	21	16	5	227
Chili, Large	12 oz	31	24	7	300
SUB SANDWICHES					
ARBYS					
French Dip	1 sandwich	42	40	2	440
Hot Ham 'n Cheese	1 sandwich	45	42	3	530
Italian	1 sandwich	49	46	3	780
Philly Beef 'n Cheese	1 sandwich	46	42	4	700
Roast Beef	1 sandwich	47	44	3	760
Turkey	1 sandwich	51	49	2	630

BLIMPIE

Cold and hot subs analyzed with 6" white sub roll w/cheese (except Seafood, Tuna, BLT, Grilled Chicken, MexiMax, ChikMax, & VegMax), lettuce, tomato, and onion. Grilled subs were prepared according to their individual specialty recipes.

FOOD	SERVING	TOTAL CARBS (G)	NET CARBS (G)	FIBER (G)	CALORIES
Blimpie Best, Cold Sub	6" regular sub	52	49.7	3.3	476
Club, Cold Sub	6" regular sub	50.5	47.3	3.3	440
Ham & Cheese, Cold Sub	6" regular sub	51.5	48.3	3.3	436
Roast Beef, Cold Sub	6" regular sub	49	45.7	3.3	468
Seafood, Cold Sub	6" regular sub	58	54.2	3.8	355
Tuna, Cold Sub	6" regular sub	50.5	47.3	3.3	493
Turkey, Cold Sub	6" regular sub	49	45.7	3.3	424
Beef, Turkey, & Cheddar, Grilled Sub	6" regular sub	49	46.3	2.7	600
Cuban, Grilled Sub	6" regular sub	50.4	47.7	2.7	462
Pastrami, Grilled Sub	6" regular sub	52	48.7	3.3	462
Reuben, Grilled Sub	6" regular sub	55	52.6	2.4	630
Ultimate Club, Grilled Sub	6" regular sub	51	48.3	2.7	724

FAST FOOD AND OTHER RESTAURANTS

FOOD	SERVING	TOTAL CARBS (G)	NET CARBS (G)	FIBER (G)	CALORIES
BLT, Hot Sub	6" regular sub	49	45.7	3.3	588
Grilled Chicken, Hot Sub	6" regular sub	50	46.7	3.3	373
Buffalo Chicken, Hot Sub	6" regular sub	50	47.3	2.7	400
Meatball, Hot Sub	6" regular sub	55	53.3	1.7	572
Pastrami, Hot Sub	6" regular sub	53	49.7	3.3	507
Steak & Onion Melt, Hot Sub	6" regular sub	49	46	3	440
MexiMax, Hot Sub	6" regular sub	65	57.7	7.3	425
ChikMax, Hot Sub	6" regular sub	71	63	8	511
VegMax, Hot Sub	6" regular sub	60	51.7	8.3	395
Durango Roast Beef & Cheddar, w/Wasabi Horseradish Sauce (from Blimpie Carb Counter Menu)	6" regular sub	na	8	na	na
Baja Turkey & Cheese w/Southwestern Chipotle Sauce (from Blimpie Carb Counter Menu)	6" regular sub	na	8	na	na
Buffalo Chicken w/Sun Dried Tomato Sauce (from Blimpie Carb Counter Menu)	6" regular sub	na	9.5	na	na
Tuscan Ham & Swiss w/Yellow Mustard (from Blimpie Carb Counter Menu)	6" regular sub	na	11	na	na
QUIZNOS					
Chicken Carbonara w/Dressing	6" sub	na	8.8	na	na

FAST FOOD AND OTHER RESTAURANTS 207

FOOD	SERVING	TOTAL CARBS (G)	NET CARBS (G)	FIBER (G)	CALORIES
Chicken Carbonara w/o Dressing	6" sub	na	5.8	na	na
Classic Italian w/Dressing	6" sub	na	10.4	na	na
Classic Italian w/o Dressing	6" sub	na	8.5	na	na
The Traditional w/Dressing	6" sub	na	12	na	na
The Traditional w/o Dressing	6" sub	na	9.9	na	na
Spicy Monterey Club w/Dressing	6" sub	na	14.9	na	na
Spicy Monterey Club w/o Dressing	6" sub	na	8.6	na	na
Honey Mustard Chicken w/Bacon w/Dressing	6" sub	na	11.4	na	na
Honey Mustard Chicken w/Bacon, w/o Dressing	6" sub	na	7.4	na	na
Mesquite Chicken w/Bacon w/Dressing	6" sub	na	9.6	na	na
Mesquite Chicken w/Bacon, w/o Dressing	6" sub	na	7.6	na	na
Honey Bacon Club w/Dressing	6" sub	na	20.3	na	na
Honey Bacon Club w/o Dressing	6" sub	na	10.3	na	na
Smoked Turkey w/Dressing	6" sub	na	11.3	na	na
Smoked Turkey w/o Dressing	6" sub	na	8.3	na	na

FAST FOOD AND OTHER RESTAURANTS

FOOD	SERVING	TOTAL CARBS (G)	NET CARBS (G)	FIBER (G)	CALORIES
Black Angus Steak w/Dressing	6" sub	na	19.2	na	na
Black Angus Steak w/o Dressing	6" sub	na	7.7	na	na
Philly Cheesesteak w/Dressing	6" sub	na	15.5	na	na
Philly Cheesesteak w/o Dressing	6" sub	na	9.5	na	na
Turkey Ranch & Swiss w/Dressing	6" sub	na	11.6	na	na
Turkey Ranch & Swiss w/o Dressing	6" sub	na	9.6	na	na
Oven Roasted Turkey	6" sub	na	8.4	na	na
Meatball	6" sub	na	9	na	na
Classic Club w/Bacon	6" sub	na	9.1	na	na
Double Cheese w/Dressing	6" sub	na	8.4	na	na
Double Cheese w/o Dressing	6" sub	na	6.4	na	na
Turkey Bacon Guac w/Dressing	6" sub	na	13.7	na	na
Turkey Bacon Guac w/o Dressing	6" sub	na	11.7	na	na
BLT w/Dressing	6" sub	na	8.7	na	na
BLT w/o Dressing	6" sub	na	6.7	na	na
Veggie w/Dressing	6" sub	na	12.2	na	na
Veggie w/o Dressing	6" sub	na	9.7	na	na
Honey Bourbon Chicken w/Dressing	6" sub	45	18.9	3	359

FAST FOOD AND OTHER RESTAURANTS

FOOD	SERVING	TOTAL CARBS (G)	NET CARBS (G)	FIBER (G)	CALORIES
Honey Bourbon Chicken w/o Dressing	6" sub	na	6.9	na	na
Sierra Smoked Turkey w/Dressing	6" sub	53	21.2	3	350
Sierra Smoked Turkey w/o Dressing	6" sub	na	7.9	na	na
Turkey Lite w/Dressing	6" sub	52	19.7	3	334
Turkey Lite w/o Dressing	6" sub	na	9.7	na	na
Ham & Swiss	6" sub	na	9.7	na	na
Tuna w/Dressing	6" sub	na	9.2	na	na
Tuna w/o Dressing	6" sub	na	7.2	na	na
Beef & Cheddar	6" sub	na	7.2	na	na
Pastrami	6" sub	na	8.1	na	na
SUBWAY (6 GRAMS OF FAT OR LESS)					
Ham*	6" sub	46	42	4	290
Roast Beef*	6" sub	45	41	4	290
Roasted Chicken Breast*	6" sub	47	42	5	320
Turkey Breast, Ham & Roast Beef Subway Club*	6" sub	46	42	4	320
Savory Turkey Breast*	6" sub	46	42	4	280
Savory Turkey Breast & Ham*	6" sub	46	42	4	290
Veggie Delite*	6" sub	44	40	4	230
Sweet Onion Chicken Teriyaki*	6" sub	59	54	5	271

* Nutrient values for Italian or wheat bread, lettuce, tomatoes, onions, green peppers, olives, and pickles.

FAST FOOD AND OTHER RESTAURANTS

FOOD	SERVING	TOTAL CARBS (G)	NET CARBS (G)	FIBER (G)	CALORIES
Honey Mustard Ham*	6" sub	54	49	5	310
Turkey Breast, Ham & Bacon Melt (Hot Sub)	6" sub	47	43	4	380
Cheese Steak (Hot Sub)	6" sub	47	42	5	360
Chipotle Southwest Cheese Steak (Hot Sub)	6" sub	49	44	5	440
Dijon Turkey Breast, Ham & Bacon Melt (Hot Sub)	6" sub	48	43	5	470
Meatball Marinara (Hot Sub)	6" sub	52	47	5	500
Classic Tuna	6" sub	46	42	4	430
Cold Cut Combo	6" sub	46	42	4	410
Italian BMT	6" sub	47	43	4	450
Subway Seafood Sensation	6" sub	52	47	5	380
Savory Turkey Breast, Deli Style	1 deli sandwich	36	33	3	210
Ham, Deli Style	1 deli sandwich	35	32	3	210
Roast Beef, Deli Style	1 deli sandwich	35	32	3	220
Classic Tuna, Deli Style	1 deli sandwich	36	33	3	300
Double Meat Turkey Breast	6" sub	48	44	4	330
Double Meat Turkey Breast & Ham	6" sub	48	44	4	360
Double Meat Ham	6" sub	49	45	4	350
Double Meat Roast Beef	6" sub	46	42	4	360

* Nutrient values for Italian or wheat bread, lettuce, tomatoes, onions, green peppers, olives, and pickles.

FAST FOOD AND OTHER RESTAURANTS

FOOD	SERVING	TOTAL CARBS (G)	NET CARBS (G)	FIBER (G)	CALORIES
Double Meat Turkey Breast, Ham & Roast Beef Club	6" sub	49	45	4	410
Double Meat Chicken	6" sub	50	45	5	430
Double Meat Classic Tuna	6" sub	48	44	4	580
Double Meat Seafood Sensation	6" sub	60	55	5	490
Double Meat Italian BMT	6" sub	49	45	4	630
Double Meat Cold Cut Combo	6" sub	48	44	4	550
Double Meat Turkey Breast, Ham & Bacon Melt (Hot Sub)	6" sub	51	47	4	490
Double Meat Cheese Steak (Hot Sub)	6" sub	50	44	6	450
Double Meat Meatball Marinara (Hot Sub)	6" sub	61	56	5	740
Double Meat Sweet Onion Chicken Teriyaki	6" sub	59	55	4	450
Double Meat Chipotle Southwest Cheese Steak (Hot Sub)	6" sub	52	46	6	530
TACOS AND OTHER MEXICAN SPECIALTIES					
JACK IN THE BOX					
Chicken Monster Taco	1 serving	18	16	2	180
Monster Taco	1 serving	20	17	3	240
Taco	1 serving	15	13	2	160

FAST FOOD AND OTHER RESTAURANTS

FOOD	SERVING	TOTAL CARBS (G)	NET CARBS (G)	FIBER (G)	CALORIES
TACO BELL					
Taco, Fresco Style*	1 serving	14	11	3	150
Soft Taco, Beef, Fresco Style*	1 serving	22	19	3	190
Soft Taco, Chicken, Fresco Style*	1 serving	20	18	2	170
Grilled Steak Soft Taco, Fresco Style*	1 serving	21	19	2	170
Gordita Baja, Beef, Fresco Style*	1 serving	30	26	4	250
Gordita Baja, Chicken, Fresco Style*	1 serving	29	27	2	230
Gordita Baja, Steak, Fresco Style*	1 serving	29	26	3	230
Bean Burrito, Fresco Style*	1 serving	56	47	9	350
Burrito Supreme, Chicken, Fresco Style*	1 serving	50	44	6	350
Burrito Supreme, Steak, Fresco Style*	1 serving	50	44	6	350
Fiesta Burrito, Chicken, Fresco Style*	1 serving	49	45	4	350
Tostada, Fresco Style*	1 serving	30	22	8	200
Enchirito, Beef, Fresco Style*	1 serving	35	28	7	270
Enchirito, Chicken, Fresco Style*	1 serving	34	29	5	250
Enchirito, Steak, Fresco Style*	1 serving	34	28	6	250

* Fresco Style items substitute Fiesta Salsa for cheese and sauce and have less than 10 grams of fat.

FOOD	SERVING	TOTAL CARBS (G)	NET CARBS (G)	FIBER (G)	CALORIES
Taco	1 serving	13	10	3	170
Taco Supreme	1 serving	14	11	3	220
Soft Taco, Beef	1 serving	21	19	2	210
Soft Taco, Chicken	1 serving	19	19	t	190
Soft Taco Supreme, Beef	1 serving	22	19	3	260
Soft Taco Supreme, Chicken	1 serving	21	20	1	230
Grilled Steak Soft Taco	1 serving	21	20	1	280
Double Decker Taco	1 serving	39	33	6	340
Double Decker Taco Supreme	1 serving	40	34	6	380
Gordita Supreme, Beef	1 serving	30	27	3	310
Gordita Supreme, Chicken	1 serving	28	26	2	290
Gordita Supreme, Steak	1 serving	28	26	2	290
Gordita Baja, Beef	1 serving	31	27	4	350
Gordita Baja, Chicken	1 serving	29	27	2	320
Gordita Baja, Steak	1 serving	29	27	2	320
Gordita Nacho Cheese, Beef	1 serving	32	29	3	300
Gordita Nacho Cheese, Chicken	1 serving	30	28	2	270
Gordita Nacho Cheese, Steak	1 serving	30	28	2	270
Chalupas Supreme, Beef	1 serving	31	28	3	390
Chalupas Supreme, Chicken	1 serving	30	29	1	370

FAST FOOD AND OTHER RESTAURANTS

FOOD	SERVING	TOTAL CARBS (G)	NET CARBS (G)	FIBER (G)	CALORIES
Chalupas Supreme, Steak	1 serving	29	27	2	370
Chalupas Baja, Beef	1 serving	32	29	3	430
Chalupas Baja, Chicken	1 serving	30	28	2	400
Chalupas Baja, Steak	1 serving	30	28	2	400
Chalupas Nacho Cheese, Beef	1 serving	33	30	3	380
Chalupas Nacho Cheese, Chicken	1 serving	31	30	1	350
Chalupas Nacho Cheese, Steak	1 serving	31	29	2	350
Bean Burrito	1 serving	55	47	8	370
7-Layer Burrito	1 serving	67	57	10	530
Chili Cheese Burrito	1 serving	40	37	3	390
Burrito Supreme, Beef	1 serving	51	44	7	440
Burrito Supreme, Chicken	1 serving	50	45	5	410
Burrito Supreme, Steak	1 serving	50	44	6	420
Fiesta Burrito, Beef	1 serving	50	45	5	390
Fiesta Burrito, Chicken	1 serving	48	45	3	370
Fiesta Burrito, Steak	1 serving	48	44	4	370
Grilled Stuft Burrito Beef	1 serving	79	69	10	730
Grilled Stuft Burrito Chicken	1 serving	76	69	7	680
Grilled Stuft Burrito Steak	1 serving	76	68	8	680
Tostada	1 serving	29	22	7	250
Mexican Pizza	1 serving	46	39	7	550
Enchirito, Beef	1 serving	35	29	6	380

FOOD	SERVING	TOTAL CARBS (G)	NET CARBS (G)	FIBER (G)	CALORIES
Enchirito, Chicken	1 serving	33	28	5	350
Enchirito, Steak	1 serving	33	28	5	360
MexiMelt	1 serving	23	20	3	290
Taco Salad w/Salsa	1 serving	73	60	13	790
Taco Salad w/Salsa & w/o Shell	1 serving	33	22	11	420
Express Taco Salad w/Chips	1 serving	60	47	13	620
Cheese Quesadilla	1 serving	39	36	3	490
Chicken Quesadilla	1 serving	40	37	3	540
Steak Quesadilla	1 serving	40	37	3	540
Zesty Chicken Border Bowl	1 serving	65	53	12	730
Zesty Chicken Border Bowl w/o Dressing	1 serving	60	48	12	500
Southwest Steak Bowl	1 serving	71	58	13	700
Nachos	1 serving	33	31	2	320
Nachos Supreme	1 serving	42	35	7	450
Nachos BellGrande	1 serving	80	68	12	780
Pintos 'n Cheese	1 serving	20	14	6	180
Mexican Rice	1 serving	23	20	3	210
Cinnamon Twists	1 serving	28	28	0	160
TACO JOHN'S					
Sierra Taco, Beef	1 serving	38	34	4	430
Sierra Taco, Chicken	1 serving	37	34	3	390
Taco Bravo	1 serving	39	31	8	340
Crispy Taco	1 serving	13	10	3	180
Softshell Taco	1 serving	21	17	4	220
Chicken Softshell	1 serving	19	15	4	190

FAST FOOD AND OTHER RESTAURANTS

FOOD	SERVING	TOTAL CARBS (G)	NET CARBS (G)	FIBER (G)	CALORIES
Taco Burger	1 serving	28	25	3	280
Super Burrito	1 serving	49	39	10	450
Meat & Potato Burrito	1 serving	55	46	9	490
Chicken & Potato Burrito	1 serving	54	46	8	460
Bean Burrito	1 serving	53	43	10	380
Beefy Burrito	1 serving	41	33	8	430
Combination Burrito	1 serving	47	38	9	400
Chicken Fiesta Salad w/o Dressing	1 serving	24	20	4	400
Taco Salad w/o Dressing	1 serving	46	42	4	580
Chicken Taco Salad w/o Dressing	1 serving	45	42	3	530
Nachos	1 serving	38	38	t	380
Super Nachos	1 serving	83	78	5	830
Chicken Super Nachos	1 serving	62	59	3	780
Potato Oles, Small	1 serving	48	43	5	440
Potato Oles, Medium	1 serving	67	61	6	620
Potato Oles, Large	1 serving	86	78	8	790
Potato Oles, Kid's Meal	1 serving	33	30	3	300
Super Potato Oles	1 serving	82	72	10	980
Pototao Oles Bravo	1 serving	55	49	6	580
Potato Oles w/Nacho Cheese	1 serving	52	47	5	550
Cheese Quesadilla	1 serving	39	33	6	480
Chicken Quesadilla	1 serving	41	34	7	540
Texas Style Chili	1 serving	26	22	4	270
Refried Beans	1 serving	50	39	11	400
Side Salad w/o Dressing	1 serving	6	5	1	80
Mexican Rice	1 serving	45	43	2	250

FAST FOOD AND OTHER RESTAURANTS

FOOD	SERVING	TOTAL CARBS (G)	NET CARBS (G)	FIBER (G)	CALORIES
Churros	1 serving	31	30	1	230
Choco Taco	1 serving	38	37	1	300
Apple Grande	1 serving	36	36	0	240
Taco John's Cookies (Kid's Meal)	1 bag	18	18	0	130
Elf Grahams (Kid's Meal)	1 bag	9	9	0	60
Taco John's Cinnamon Mint Swirl	1 serving	3	3	0	10

WRAPS

ARBY'S

Market Fresh Low Carbys LTO Items (Limited Time Only)

These items may be available only at participating Arby's franchises.

FOOD	SERVING	TOTAL CARBS (G)	NET CARBS (G)	FIBER (G)	CALORIES
Market Fresh Low Carbys Wrap Roast Turkey Ranch & Bacon	1 wrap	50	18	32	710
Market Fresh Low Carbys Wrap Ultimate BLT	1 wrap	50	17	33	660

BLIMPIE

FOOD	SERVING	TOTAL CARBS (G)	NET CARBS (G)	FIBER (G)	CALORIES
Chicken Caesar	1 wrap, regular	56	53	3	646
Beef & Cheddar	1 wrap, regular	57	54	3	714
Southwestern	1 wrap, regular	54	51	3	674
Steak & Onions	1 wrap, regular	64	61	3	716
Ultimate BLT	1 wrap, regular	60	57	3	831
Zesty Italian	1 wrap, regular	74	71	3	638

CHICK-FIL-A

FOOD	SERVING	TOTAL CARBS (G)	NET CARBS (G)	FIBER (G)	CALORIES
Chargrilled Chicken Cool Wraps	1 wrap (8.63 g)	54	51	3	380

FOOD	SERVING	TOTAL CARBS (G)	NET CARBS (G)	FIBER (G)	CALORIES
Chicken Caesar Cool Wrap	1 wrap (8 g)	52	50	2	460
Spicy Chicken Cool Wrap	1 wrap (8.13 g)	52	49	3	380
RUBY TUESDAY					
Black & Bleu Burger Wrap, Low Carb	1 wrap	na	12	10	793
Burger Wrap, Low Carb	1 wrap	na	7	10	624
Peppercorn Chicken Caesar Wrap, Low Carb	1 wrap	na	16	11	494
Pepper Jack Burger Wrap, Low Carb	1 wrap	na	12	10	864
Roasted Turkey Wrap, Low Carb	1 wrap	na	10	11	346
Spicy Chicken Wrap	1 wrap	na	10	10	475
Turkey Burger Club Wrap, Low Carb	1 wrap	na	8	10	574
Turkey Burger Wrap, Low Carb	1 wrap	na	8	10	426
SCHLOTZSKY'S DELI					
Asian Almond Chicken	1 wrap	72	68	4	459
Salsa Chicken w/Cheddar	1 wrap	44	41	3	460
Zesty Albacore Tuna	1 wrap	45	42	3	311
Chicken Caesar	1 wrap	40	37	3	511
SONIC					
Grilled Chicken Wrap	1 wrap	40	38	2	539

FOOD	SERVING	TOTAL CARBS (G)	NET CARBS (G)	FIBER (G)	CALORIES
Grilled Chicken Wrap w/o Ranch dressing	1 wrap	38	36	2	393
Chicken Strip Wrap	1 wrap	55	53	2	574
Chicken Strip Wrap w/o Ranch dressing	1 wrap	53	51	2	428
Fritos Chili Cheese Wrap	1 wrap	68	63	5	743
SUBWAY					
Chicken Bacon Ranch w/Swiss Cheese	1 wrap	17	8	9	440
Turkey Bacon Melt w/Monterey Cheddar Cheese	1 wrap	20	11	9	430
Turkey Breast & Ham	1 wrap	19	10	9	390
T.G.I. FRIDAY'S					
Tuna Salad Wraps	1 serving	na	14	na	na

FATS AND OILS

BUTTER

FOOD	SERVING	TOTAL CARBS (G)	NET CARBS (G)	FIBER (G)	CALORIES
Butter, light, stick w/salt	1 tsp	0	0	0	69
Butter, whipped, w/salt	1 pat (1" sq x ⅓" high)	0	0	0	27
Butter, w/salt	1 pat (1" sq x ⅓" high)	0	0	0	36

MARGARINE AND SPREADS

FOOD	SERVING	TOTAL CARBS (G)	NET CARBS (G)	FIBER (G)	CALORIES
Margarine, 80% fat, stick, includes regular & hydrogenated corn & soybean oils	1 tsp	0	0	0	33

220 FATS AND OILS

FOOD	SERVING	TOTAL CARBS (G)	NET CARBS (G)	FIBER (G)	CALORIES
Margarine, 70% vegetable oil spread, soybean (hydrogenated)	1 tsp	0	0	0	29
Margarine, regular, hard, coconut (hydrogenated & regular) & safflower & palm (hydrogenated)	1 tsp	0	0	0	34
Margarine, regular, hard, corn (hydrogenated & regular)	1 tsp	0	0	0	34
Margarine, regular, hard, corn (hydrogenated)	1 tsp	0	0	0	34
Margarine, regular, hard, corn & soybean (hydrogenated) & cottonseed (hydrogenated), w/salt	1 tsp	0	0	0	34
Margarine, regular, hard, corn & soybean (hydrogenated) & cottonseed (hydrogenated), w/o salt	1 tsp	0	0	0	34
Margarine, regular, hard, lard (hydrogenated)	1 tsp	0	0	0	34

FATS AND OILS 221

FOOD	SERVING	TOTAL CARBS (G)	NET CARBS (G)	FIBER (G)	CALORIES
Margarine, regular, hard, safflower & soybean (hydrogenated & regular) & cottonseed (hydrogenated)	1 tsp	0	0	0	34
Margarine, regular, hard, safflower & soybean (hydrogenated)	1 tsp	0	0	0	34
Margarine, regular, hard, safflower & soybean (hydrogenated) & cottonseed (hydrogenated)	1 tsp	0	0	0	34
Margarine, regular, hard, soybean (hydrogenated & regular)	1 tsp	0	0	0	34
Margarine, regular, hard, soybean (hydrogenated)	1 tsp	0	0	0	34
Margarine, regular, liquid, soybean (hydrogenated & regular) & cottonseed	1 tsp	0	0	0	34
Margarine, regular, unspecified oils, w/salt	1 tsp	0	0	0	34

FATS AND OILS

FOOD	SERVING	TOTAL CARBS (G)	NET CARBS (G)	FIBER (G)	CALORIES
Margarine, regular, unspecified oils, w/o salt	1 tsp	0	0	0	34
Margarine, soft, corn (hydrogenated & regular)	1 tsp	0	0	0	34
Margarine, soft, safflower (hydrogenated & regular)	1 tsp	0	0	0	34
Margarine, soft, soybean (hydrogenated & regular), w/salt	1 tsp	0	0	0	34
Margarine, soft, soybean (hydrogenated) & safflower	1 tsp	0	0	0	34
Margarine-butter blend, 60% corn oil margarine & 40% butter	1 tsp	t	t	0	34
Margarinelike spread, approx. 40% fat, corn (hydrogenated & regular)	1 tsp	t	t	0	17
Margarinelike spread, approx. 40% fat, soybean (hydrogenated)	1 tsp	t	t	0	17
Margarinelike spread, approx. 40% fat, unspecified oils	1 tsp	t	t	0	17

FATS AND OILS

FOOD	SERVING	TOTAL CARBS (G)	NET CARBS (G)	FIBER (G)	CALORIES
Margarinelike spread, approx. 60% fat, stick, soybean (hydrogenated & regular)	1 tsp	0	0	0	26
Margarinelike spread, approx. 60% fat, tub, unspecified oils	1 tsp	0	0	0	26
Shortening, multipurpose, soybean (hydrogenated) & palm (hydrogenated)	1 tbsp	0	0	0	113
Shortening, household, soybean (hydrogenated) & palm	1 tbsp	0	0	0	113
Shortening, household, soybean (hydrogenated) & cottonseed (hydrogenated)	1 tbsp	0	0	0	113
STICKS, BY BRAND					
Fleischmann's Light Margarine	1 tbsp	0	0	na	50
Parkay Light Stick	1 tbsp	0	0	na	50
Promise Buttery Light	1 tbsp	0	0	na	50
Promise Spread	1 tbsp	0	0	na	90
SPRAYS, PUMPS & BOTTLED OILS					
I Can't Believe It's Not Butter! Spray	5 sprays	0	0	0	0
Pam & Similar Vegetable Sprays	1 spray	0	0	na	7
Keto Butta (Natural Butter Flavored MCT Oil)	1 tbsp	0	0	0	43

FATS AND OILS

FOOD	SERVING	TOTAL CARBS (G)	NET CARBS (G)	FIBER (G)	CALORIES
Keto High Oleic Sunflower Oil	1 tbsp	0	0	0	130
TUBS AND SQUEEZE BOTTLES					
Benecol Spread	1 tbsp	0	0	na	80
Benecol Light Spread	1 tbsp	0	0	na	45
Blue Bonnet Home Style Spread	1 tbsp	0	0	na	60
Brummel & Brown Spread w/Yogurt	1 tbsp	0	0	0	45
Canoleo Margarine	1 tbsp	0	0	0	100
Earth Balance Natural Buttery Spread	1 tbsp	0	0	na	100
Fleischmann's Light Margarine	1 tbsp	0	0	na	40
Fleischmann's Original Spread	1 tbsp	0	0	na	80
Fleischmann's Premium Spread w/Olive Oil	1 tbsp	0	0	na	70
Fleischmann's Unsalted Spread	1 tbsp	0	0	na	80
I Can't Believe It's Not Butter! Fat Free Spread	1 tbsp	0	0	0	5
I Can't Believe It's Not Butter! Light Spread	1 tbsp	0	0	0	50
I Can't Believe It's Not Butter! Sweet Cream & Calcium Spread	1 tbsp	0	0	0	50
Olivio Premium Spread w/Olive Oil	1 tbsp	0	0	na	80
Parkay Calcium Plus Spread	1 tbsp	0	0	na	45

FATS AND OILS   225

FOOD	SERVING	TOTAL CARBS (G)	NET CARBS (G)	FIBER (G)	CALORIES
Parkay Light Spread	1 tbsp	0	0	na	50
Parkay Spread	1 tbsp	0	0	na	80
Parkay Squeeze Spread	1 tbsp	0	0	na	70
Promise Buttery Light Spread	1 tbsp	0	0	0	50
Promise Fat Free Spread	1 tbsp	0	0	0	5
Promise Spread	1 tbsp	0	0	0	80
Promise Ultra	1 tbsp	0	0	0	40
Smart Balance Buttery Spread	1 tbsp	0	0	0	80
Smart Balance Light Spread	1 tbsp	0	0	0	50
Smart Beat Fat Free Squeeze Margarine	1 tbsp	0	0	0	5
Smart Beat Trans Free Super Light Margarine	1 tbsp	0	0	0	20
Smart Beat Unsalted Light Margarine	1 tbsp	0	0	0	30
Shedd's Spread Churn Style Country Crock	1 tbsp	0	0	0	60
Shedd's Spread Country Crock Easy Squeeze	1 tbsp	0	0	0	60
Shedd's Spread Country Crock Plus Calcium & Vitamins	1 tbsp	0	0	0	50
Shedd's Spread Light Country Crock	1 tbsp	0	0	0	50
Take Control Spread	1 tbsp	0	0	0	80
Take Control Light Spread	1 tbsp	0	0	0	45

FATS AND OILS

FOOD	SERVING	TOTAL CARBS (G)	NET CARBS (G)	FIBER (G)	CALORIES
MISCELLANEOUS FATS					
Bacon grease	1 tsp	0	0	0	38
Beef tallow	1 tbsp	0	0	0	115
Lard	1 tbsp	0	0	0	115
OILS					
Almond oil	1 tbsp	0	0	0	119
Apricot kernel oil	1 tbsp	0	0	0	119
Avocado oil	1 tbsp	0	0	0	124
Butter replacement, w/o fat, powder	1 tsp	1	1	0	6
Canola oil	1 tbsp	0	0	0	124
Coconut oil	1 tbsp	0	0	0	116
Corn oil, salad or cooking	1 tbsp	0	0	0	120
Flaxseed oil	1 tbsp	0	0	0	119
Grapeseed oil	1 tbsp	0	0	0	120
Hazelnut nut oil	1 tbsp	0	0	0	119
Olive oil, salad or cooking	1 tbsp	0	0	0	119
Peanut oil, salad or cooking	1 tbsp	0	0	0	119
Sesame oil, salad or cooking	1 tbsp	0	0	0	120
Safflower oil (70% linoleic), salad or cooking	1 tbsp	0	0	0	120
Safflower oil (over 70% safflower) salad or cooking	1 tbsp	0	0	0	120

FOOD	SERVING	TOTAL CARBS (G)	NET CARBS (G)	FIBER (G)	CALORIES
Soybean oil, salad or cooking	1 tbsp	0	0	0	120
Sunflower oil (less than 60% linoleic)	1 tbsp	0	0	0	120
Sunflower oil (more than 60% linoleic)	1 tbsp	0	0	0	120
Sunflower oil (more than 70% oleic)	1 tbsp	0	0	0	124
Walnut oil	1 tbsp	0	0	0	120
Wheat germ oil	1 tbsp	0	0	0	120

FISH AND SHELLFISH

FISH

FOOD	SERVING	TOTAL CARBS (G)	NET CARBS (G)	FIBER (G)	CALORIES
Anchovy, canned in oil, drained	1 can (2 oz)	0	0	0	95
Bass, freshwater, mixed species, cooked	4 oz	0	0	0	165
Bass, striped, cooked	4 oz	0	0	0	141
Bluefish, cooked	4 oz	0	0	0	180
Burbot, cooked	4 oz	0	0	0	130
Butterfish, cooked	4 oz	0	0	0	212
Carp, cooked	4 oz	0	0	0	184
Catfish, breaded & fried	4 oz	9	8	1	260
Catfish, channel, farmed, cooked	4 oz	0	0	0	172
Catfish, channel, wild, cooked	4 oz	0	0	0	119
Caviar, black & red, granular	3 tbsp	2	2	0	121
Cod, Atlantic, canned	4 oz	0	0	0	119

FISH AND SHELLFISH

FOOD	SERVING	TOTAL CARBS (G)	NET CARBS (G)	FIBER (G)	CALORIES
Cod, Atlantic, cooked	4 oz	0	0	0	119
Cod, Pacific, cooked	4 oz	0	0	0	119
Croaker, breaded & fried	4 oz	9	8.5	.5	250
Dolphinfish, cooked	4 oz	0	0	0	124
Drum, freshwater, cooked	4 oz	0	0	0	173
Fish fillet, fried, generic	1 fillet	15.5	15	.5	211
Fish sticks, frozen, preheated	4 sticks	27	27	0	305
Flounder, cooked	4 oz	0	0	0	133
Grouper, mixed species, cooked	4 oz	0	0	0	134
Haddock, cooked	4 oz	0	0	0	127
Halibut, Atlantic & Pacific, cooked	4 oz	0	0	0	159
Halibut, Greenland, cooked	4 oz	0	0	0	271
Herring, Atlantic, cooked	4 oz	0	0	0	230
Herring, Atlantic, kippered, large (7" x 2¼" x ¼")	1 fillet	0	0	0	141
Herring, Atlantic, pickled, (1¾" x ⅞" x ½")	3 pieces	4	4	0	118
Herring, Pacific, cooked	4 oz	0	0	0	283
Mackerel, Atlantic, cooked	4 oz	0	0	0	297

FOOD	SERVING	TOTAL CARBS (G)	NET CARBS (G)	FIBER (G)	CALORIES
Mackerel, jack, canned, boneless	4 oz	0	0	0	177
Mackerel, king, cooked	4 oz	0	0	0	152
Mackerel, Pacific & jack, mixed species, cooked, boneless	4 oz	0	0	0	228
Mackerel, Spanish, cooked	4 oz	0	0	0	179
Monkfish, cooked	4 oz	0	0	0	110
Mullet, striped, cooked	4 oz	0	0	0	170
Ocean perch, Atlantic, cooked	4 oz	0	0	0	137
Orange roughy, cooked	4 oz	0	0	0	101
Perch, mixed species, cooked	4 oz	0	0	0	133
Pike, northern, cooked	4 oz	0	0	0	128
Pike, walleye, cooked	4 oz	0	0	0	135
Pollock, Atlantic, cooked	4 oz	0	0	0	134
Pollock, walleye, cooked	4 oz	0	0	0	128
Pompano, Florida, cooked	4 oz	0	0	0	239
Rockfish, Pacific, mixed species, cooked	4 oz	0	0	0	137
Roe, mixed species, cooked	4 oz	2	2	0	231
Salmon, Atlantic, farmed, cooked	4 oz	0	0	0	233

230 FISH AND SHELLFISH

FOOD	SERVING	TOTAL CARBS (G)	NET CARBS (G)	FIBER (G)	CALORIES
Salmon, Atlantic, wild, cooked	4 oz	0	0	0	206
Salmon, Chinook, cooked	4 oz	0	0	0	262
Salmon, Chinook, smoked (lox), cooked	4 oz	0	0	0	133
Salmon, chum, cooked	4 oz	0	0	0	175
Salmon, chum, drained solids, w/bone	4 oz	0	0	0	160
Salmon, coho, farmed, cooked	4 oz	0	0	0	202
Salmon, coho, wild, cooked	4 oz	0	0	0	158
Salmon, pink, canned, solids w/ bone & liquid	4 oz	0	0	0	158
Salmon, pink, cooked	4 oz	0	0	0	169
Salmon, sockeye, canned, drained solids w/bone	4 oz	0	0	0	173
Salmon, sockeye, cooked	4 oz	0	0	0	245
Salmon, smoked					
Sardine, canned in oil, drained	4 oz	0	0	0	236
Sardines, Pacific, canned in tomato sauce, drained solids w/bone	3 pieces	0	0	0	203

FISH AND SHELLFISH

FOOD	SERVING	TOTAL CARBS (G)	NET CARBS (G)	FIBER (G)	CALORIES
Sea bass, mixed species, cooked	4 oz	0	0	0	141
Sea trout, mixed species, cooked	4 oz	0	0	0	151
Shad, American, cooked	4 oz	0	0	0	286
Shark	4 oz	0	0	0	147
Shark, breaded & fried	4 oz	7	7	0	258
Smelt, rainbow, cooked	4 oz	0	0	0	141
Snapper, mixed species, cooked	4 oz	0	0	0	145
Spot, cooked	4 oz	0	0	0	179
Sturgeon, mixed species, cooked, boneless	4 oz	0	0	0	153
Sunfish, pumpkin seed, cooked	4 oz	0	0	0	129
Surimi	4 oz	8	8	0	112
Swordfish, cooked	4 oz	0	0	0	176
Tilefish, cooked	4 oz	0	0	0	167
Trout, mixed species, cooked	4 oz	0	0	0	215
Trout, rainbow, farmed, cooked	4 oz	0	0	0	192
Trout, rainbow, wild, cooked	4 oz	0	0	0	170
Tuna, bluefin, fresh, cooked	4 oz	0	0	0	209

FISH AND SHELLFISH

FOOD	SERVING	TOTAL CARBS (G)	NET CARBS (G)	FIBER (G)	CALORIES
Tuna, light, canned in oil, drained	4 oz	0	0	0	225
Tuna, white, canned in oil, drained	4 oz	0	0	0	211
Tuna, light, canned in water, drained solids	4 oz	0	0	0	132
Tuna, white, canned in water, drained solids	4 oz	0	0	0	145
Tuna, yellowfish, fresh, cooked	4 oz	0	0	0	158
Turbot, European, cooked	4 oz	0	0	0	138
Whitefish, mixed species, cooked	4 oz	0	0	0	195
Whiting, mixed species, cooked	4 oz	0	0	0	131
Yellowtail, mixed species, cooked	4 oz	0	0	0	212
SHELLFISH					
Clams, breaded & fried	4 oz	12	12	na	229
Clams, mixed species, canned, drained solids	4 oz	6	2/t	0	168
Clams, mixed species, cooked	4 oz	6	2/t	0	168
Crab, Alaska King, cooked	4 oz	0	2/t	0	110
Crab, Alaska King, imitation, made from surimi	4 oz	12	1/t	0	116
Crab, blue, cooked	4 oz	0	2/t	0	116

FISH AND SHELLFISH 233

FOOD	SERVING	TOTAL CARBS (G)	NET CARBS (G)	FIBER (G)	CALORIES
Crab cakes, fried	2 cakes	.5	13	0	186
Crab, Dungeness, cooked	4 oz	1	1	0	125
Crab, Queen, cooked	4 oz	0	0	0	130
Lobster, northern, cooked	4 oz	1	1	0	111
Lobster, spiny, mixed species, cooked	4 oz	4	4	0	162
Oysters, breaded & fried	4 oz	13	13	na	223
Oyster, eastern, canned, drained	4 oz	4	4	0	63
Oyster, eastern, farmed, cooked, dry heat	4 oz	8	8	0	90
Oyster, eastern, wild, cooked, dry heat	4 oz	5	5	0	82
Oyster, eastern, wild, cooked, moist heat	4 oz	9	9	0	155
Oyster, Pacific, cooked, moist heat	4 oz	11	11	0	185
Scallop, breaded & fried	4 oz	11	11	na	241
Scallop, mixed species, imitation, made from surimi	4 oz	12	12	0	112
Shrimp, breaded & fried	4 oz	13	12.5	.5	274
Shrimp, mixed species, canned	1 oz	0	0	0	34
Shrimp, mixed species, cooked, moist heat	4 oz	0	0	0	112

FROSTINGS AND TOPPINGS

FOOD	SERVING	TOTAL CARBS (G)	NET CARBS (G)	FIBER (G)	CALORIES
Shrimp, mixed species, imitation, made from surimi	4 oz	10	10	0	114
Squid, fried (calamari)	4 oz	9	9	0	198

FROSTINGS AND TOPPINGS
FROSTINGS, BY BRAND, LOW CARB

FOOD	SERVING	TOTAL CARBS (G)	NET CARBS (G)	FIBER (G)	CALORIES
Atkins Celebration Cake Icing Kit, All Flavors	1 serving (7 g)	2	t	na	32
Atkins Whip It Up Flavoring Packets (for Frostings), Chocolate*	3 tbsp	4	4	0	2
Atkins Whip It Up Flavoring Packets (for Frostings), Strawberry*	3 tbsp	4	4	0	2
Atkins Whip It Up Flavoring Packets (for Frostings), Vanilla*	3 tbsp	4	4	0	2

FROSTINGS, GENERIC

FOOD	SERVING	TOTAL CARBS (G)	NET CARBS (G)	FIBER (G)	CALORIES
Chocolate, ready-to-eat	2 tbsp	26	26	t	163
Coconut nut, ready-to-eat	2 tbsp	19	18.5	.5	151
Cream cheese flavor, ready-to-eat	2 tbsp	22	22	0	137
Vanilla, ready-to-eat	2 tbsp	26	26	0	159

TOPPINGS, BY BRAND, LOW CARB

FOOD	SERVING	TOTAL CARBS (G)	NET CARBS (G)	FIBER (G)	CALORIES
Dixie Diners' Club Whipped Topping Mix, Chocolate	3 tbsp	0	0	0	85

* Nutrient count only for mix ingredients. Does not include Quick Whip or cream ingredients.

FROSTINGS AND TOPPINGS

FOOD	SERVING	TOTAL CARBS (G)	NET CARBS (G)	FIBER (G)	CALORIES
Dixie Diners' Club Whipped Topping Mix, Strawberry	3 tbsp	0	0	0	84
Dixie Diners' Club Whipped Topping Mix, Vanilla	3 tbsp	0	0	0	84
DaVinci Gourmet Sugar Free Chocolate Sauce	2 tbsp	5	1	t	15
Steel's Amaretto Fudge Sauce	2 tbsp	10	2	1	65
Steel's Butterscotch Sauce	2 tbsp	10	0	0	40
Steel's Caramel Sauce	2 tbsp	3	0	1	90
Steel's Chocolate Fudge Sauce	2 tbsp	5	1	2	45
Steel's Crimson Strawberry Sauce	2 tbsp	6	0	0	20
Steel's Grand Marnier Fudge Sauce	2 tbsp	10	2	1	65
Steel's Mango Curry Sauce	1 tbsp	2.8	2.5	.3	13
Steel's Peanut Butter Fudge Sauce	2 tbsp	4.5	1.5	2	75
Steel's Praline Sauce	2 tbsp	10	1	0	25
Steel's Raspberry Jalapeño Sauce	2 tbsp	1.9	.6	t	9
TOPPINGS					
Dessert topping, frozen	½ cup	8	8	0	119
Dessert topping, pressurized	½ cup	5.5	5.5	0	92

FOOD	SERVING	TOTAL CARBS (G)	NET CARBS (G)	FIBER (G)	CALORIES
Dessert topping, powdered, prepared w/½ cup milk	½ cup	6.5	6.5	0	75
Butterscotch or caramel topping	2 tbsp	27	27	t	103
Marshmallow cream topping	¼ jar	39	39	0	159
Nuts in syrup topping	2 tbsp	22	21	1	167
Pineapple topping	2 tbsp	28	28	t	106
Strawberry topping	2 tbsp	28	28	t	107

FRUITS AND FRUIT JUICES

FRUITS

FOOD	SERVING	TOTAL CARBS (G)	NET CARBS (G)	FIBER (G)	CALORIES
Acerola (West Indian cherry), raw	1 cup	8	7	1	31
Apple, dehydrated, sulfured, uncooked	½ cup	28	24	4	104
Apple, dried, sulfured, uncooked	5 rings	21	18	3	78
Apple, raw (2¾" dia), w/skin	1 fruit	21	17	4	81
Apple, raw (2¾" dia), w/o skin	1 fruit	19	17	2	73
Apple, raw, w/skin, sliced	1 cup	17	15	3	65
Apple, raw, w/o skin, sliced	1 cup	16	14	2	63
Applesauce, canned, sweetened, w/salt	½ cup	25	23.5	1.5	97
Applesauce, canned, sweetened, w/o salt	½ cup	25	23.5	1.5	97

FRUITS AND FRUIT JUICES

FOOD	SERVING	TOTAL CARBS (G)	NET CARBS (G)	FIBER (G)	CALORIES
Applesauce, unsweetened	½ cup	14	12.5	1.5	52
Apricot, canned, water pack, w/o skin	½ cup	6	5	1	25
Apricot, canned, water pack, w/skin	½ cup	8	6	2	33
Apricots, canned, extra heavy syrup, w/o skin, solids & liquids	½ cup, whole, w/o pits	31	29	2	118
Apricots, canned, heavy syrup, w/o skin, solids & liquids	½ cup, whole, w/o pits	28	26	2	107
Apricots, canned, light syrup, w/skin, solids & liquids	½ cup, halves	21	19	2	80
Apricot, dried, sulfured, uncooked	10 halves	22	19.5	2.5	84
Apricot, raw	2 fruits	8	6	2	140
Apricot, raw, sliced	1 cup	18	14	4	79
Avocado, raw, all varieties	¼ fruit	4	1.5	2.5	81
Avocado, raw, w/o skin & seeds, California	¼ fruit	3	1	2	77
Avocado, raw, w/o skin & seeds, Florida	¼ fruit	7	3	4	85
Banana (7"–7⅞" long), raw	1 fruit	28	25	3	109
Blueberries, frozen, sweetened	1 cup, thawed	50	45	5	186

FRUITS AND FRUIT JUICES

FOOD	SERVING	TOTAL CARBS (G)	NET CARBS (G)	FIBER (G)	CALORIES
Blackberries, frozen, unsweetened, unthawed	1 cup	24	16.5	7.5	97
Blackberries, raw	1 cup	18	10	8	75
Blueberries, frozen, unsweetened, unthawed	1 cup	19	14.8	4.2	79
Blueberries, raw	1 cup	20	16	4	81
Candied fruit	100 g	83	81	2	321
Cherries, sour, red, canned, in heavy syrup, solids & liquids	½ cup	30	29	1	117
Cherries, sour, red, canned, water pack	1 cup	22	19	3	88
Cherries, sour, red, frozen, unsweetened, unthawed	1 cup	17	14.5	2.5	71
Cherries, sour, red, raw, w/o pits	1 cup	19	16.5	2.5	78
Cherries, sour, red, raw, w/pits	1 cup	13	11.5	1.5	52
Cherries, sweet, canned, juice pack, pitted	1 cup	35	31	4	135
Cherries, sweet, canned, water pack, pitted	1 cup	29	25	4	114
Cherries, sweet, raw, w/o pits	1 cup	24	21	3	104
Cherries, sweet, raw, w/pits	1 cup	19	18	3	84

FRUITS AND FRUIT JUICES

FOOD	SERVING	TOTAL CARBS (G)	NET CARBS (G)	FIBER (G)	CALORIES
Cranberries, raw, chopped	1 cup	14	9.4	4.6	54
Cranberries, raw, whole	1 cup	12	8	4	47
Cranberry sauce, canned, sweetened	½ cup	54	53	1	209
Currants, black, raw	1 cup	18	18	na	71
Currants, red & white, raw	1 cup	15	10	5	63
Dates, domestic, natural & dry	5 dates	31	29	3	114
Figs, canned, water pack	½ cup	17	14	3	66
Figs, dried, stewed	½ cup	36	29	7	140
Figs, dried, uncooked	2 figs	25	20	5	97
Figs, raw, large (2½" dia)	2 figs	25	21	4	95
Fruit cocktail, canned, extra heavy syrup, solids & liquids	½ cup	30	29	1	114
Fruit cocktail, canned, heavy syrup, solids & liquids	½ cup	23	22	1	91
Fruit cocktail, canned, light syrup, solids & liquids	½ cup	18	17	1	69
Fruit salad, canned, extra heavy syrup, solids & liquids	½ cup	30	29	1	114

240 FRUITS AND FRUIT JUICES

FOOD	SERVING	TOTAL CARBS (G)	NET CARBS (G)	FIBER (G)	CALORIES
Fruit salad, canned, heavy syrup, solids & liquids	½ cup	29	27	2	111
Fruit salad, canned, light syrup, solids & liquids	½ cup	19	18	1	73
Fruit cocktail, canned, juice pack	½ cup	14	13	1	55
Fruit cocktail, canned, water pack	½ cup	10	9	1	38
Grapefruit sections, canned, in light syrup, solids & liquids	½ cup	20	19	1	76
Grapefruit, pink, raw, red & white (4" dia)	½ fruit	10	8.6	1.4	41
Grapefruit, canned sections, juice pack	½ cup	11	10.5	0.5	46
Grapefruit, canned sections, water pack	½ cup	11	10.5	0.5	44
Grapes, American, slip skin, raw	1 cup	16	15	1	62
Grapes, European, red or green, Thompson seedless, raw	1 cup	28	26.5	1.5	114
Grapes, Thompson seedless, canned, in heavy syrup, solids & liquids	½ cup	25	24.5	.5	93

FRUITS AND FRUIT JUICES

FOOD	SERVING	TOTAL CARBS (G)	NET CARBS (G)	FIBER (G)	CALORIES
Grapes, canned, Thompson seedless, water pack	½ cup	13	12	1	49
Guava, common, raw, w/o refuse	1 fruit	11	6	5	46
Kiwi fruit, fresh, raw, w/o skin, large	1 fruit	14	11	3	56
Lemon, raw, w/o peel	1 fruit (2⅜" dia)	8	5.5	2.5	24
Lemon, raw, with, w/o seeds, peel	1 fruit (2⅜" dia)	12	7	5	22
Lime, raw	1 fruit (2" dia)	7	5	2	20
Mango, raw, sliced	1 cup	28	25	3	107
Melon balls, frozen, unthawed	1 cup	14	13	1	57
Melon, cantaloupe, raw, wedge	1 wedge (⅛ of large melon)	9	8	1	36
Melon, casaba, raw, wedge	1 wedge (⅛ of melon)	13	11	2	53
Melon, honeydew, raw, wedge	1 wedge (⅛ of 6"–7" dia melon)	15	14	1	56
Nectarine, raw	1 fruit (2½" dia)	16	14	2	67
Orange, raw, California, navel	1 fruit (2⅞" dia)	16	12.5	3.5	64
Orange, raw, California, valencia	1 fruit (2⅝" dia)	14	11	3	59
Orange, raw, Florida	1 fruit (2⅝" dia)	16	12.5	3.5	65
Papaya, raw, cubes	1 cup	14	11.5	2.5	55
Papaya, raw, small	1 fruit (4½" long x 2¾" dia)	15	12	3	59

FRUITS AND FRUIT JUICES

FOOD	SERVING	TOTAL CARBS (G)	NET CARBS (G)	FIBER (G)	CALORIES
Peaches, canned, extra heavy syrup, solids & liquids	½ cup, halves or slices	34	33	1	126
Peaches, canned, heavy syrup, solids & liquids	½ cup	26	24	2	97
Peaches, canned, light syrup, solids & liquids	½ cup, halves or slices	18	16	2	68
Peaches, canned, extra light syrup, solids & liquids	½ cup, halves or slices	14	13	1	52
Peaches, spiced, canned, extra heavy syrup, solids & liquids	½ cup, whole	24	22	2	91
Peaches, canned, juice pack, halves or slices	½ cup	14	12.5	1.5	55
Peaches, canned, water pack, halves or slices	½ cup	7	5.5	1.5	29
Peaches, dried, sulfured, stewed, w/o added sugar	½ cup	25	21.5	3.5	99
Peaches, dried, sulfured, uncooked, halves	3	24	21	3	93
Peaches, raw, large	1 fruit (2¾" dia)	17	14	3	68
Peaches, raw, slices	1 cup	19	16	3	73
Pears, Asian, raw	1 fruit (2¼" long x 2½" dia)	13	9	4	51
Pears, canned, extra heavy syrup, solids & liquids	½ cup, halves	34	32	2	129

FRUITS AND FRUIT JUICES

FOOD	SERVING	TOTAL CARBS (G)	NET CARBS (G)	FIBER (G)	CALORIES
Pears, canned, heavy syrup, solids & liquids	½ cup	26	24	2	98
Pears, canned, light syrup, solids & liquids	½ cup, halves	19	17	2	72
Pears, canned, extra light syrup, solids & liquids	½ cup, halves	15	13	2	58
Pears, canned, juice pack, halves	½ cup	16	14	2	62
Pears, canned, water pack, halves	½ cup	10	8	2	35
Pear, raw, medium	1 fruit (approx. 2½ per lb)	25	21	4	98
Persimmons, Japanese, raw	1 fruit (2½" dia)	31	25	6	118
Persimmons, native, raw, w/o refuse	1 fruit	8	8	na	32
Pineapple, canned, juice pack, chunks, crushed, slices	½ cup	20	19	1	75
Pineapple, canned, extra heavy syrup, solids & liquids	½ cup, crushed, sliced or chunks	28	27	1	108
Pineapple, canned, heavy syrup, solids & liquids	½ cup, crushed, sliced or chunks	26	25	1	99
Pineapple, canned, light syrup, solids & liquids	½ cup, crushed, sliced or chunks	17	16	1	66

FRUITS AND FRUIT JUICES

FOOD	SERVING	TOTAL CARBS (G)	NET CARBS (G)	FIBER (G)	CALORIES
Pineapple, canned, water pack, chunks crushed, slices	½ cup	10	9	1	39
Pineapple, frozen, chunks, sweetened	½ cup, chunks	27	26	1	104
Pineapple, raw, diced	1 cup	19	17	2	76
Plantains, cooked, slices	½ cup	24	22	2	89
Plantains, raw, medium	½ fruit	29	27	2	109
Plums, canned, purple, extra heavy syrup, solids & liquids	½ cup, pitted	34	33	1	132
Plums, canned, purple, heavy syrup, solids & liquids	½ cup, pitted	30	29	1	115
Plums, canned, purple, light syrup, solids & liquids	½ cup, pitted	21	20	1	79
Plums, canned, purple, juice pack, pitted	½ cup	19	18	1	73
Plums, canned, purple, water pack, pitted	½ cup	14	13	1	51
Plum, raw	1 fruit (2⅛" dia)	9	8	1	36
Pomegranate, raw	1 fruit (3⅜" dia)	26	25	1	105
Prunes, canned, heavy syrup, solids & liquids	½ cup	33	29	4	123
Prunes, dried, stewed, w/added sugar	½ cup, pitted	41	36	5	154
Prunes, dried, stewed, w/o added sugar, pitted	½ cup	35	27	8	133

FRUITS AND FRUIT JUICES

FOOD	SERVING	TOTAL CARBS (G)	NET CARBS (G)	FIBER (G)	CALORIES
Prunes, dried, uncooked	5 fruits	26	23	3	100
Raisins, golden seedless, not packed	¼ cup	29	27.5	1.5	109
Raisins, seedless, not packed	¼ cup	29	27.5	1.5	109
Raisins, seedless, 5 oz miniature box	1 box	11	10	1	42
Raspberries, raw	1 cup	14	5.6	8.4	60
Rhubarb, frozen, cooked, w/sugar	½ cup	37	35	2	139
Rhubarb, frozen, uncooked, diced	1 cup	7	4.5	2.5	29
Rhubarb, raw, diced	1 cup	6	4	2	26
Strawberries, frozen, sweetened, whole	1 cup	54	49	5	199
Strawberries, frozen, unsweetened, thawed	1 cup	20	15	5	77
Strawberries, raw, sliced	1 cup	12	8	4	50
Tangerine (mandarin), canned, juice pack	½ cup	12	11	1	46
Tangerine (mandarin), raw, large	1 fruit (2½" dia)	11	9	2	43
Watermelon, raw, diced	1 cup	11	10	1	49
Watermelon, raw, wedge	1 wedge (1/16 of melon)	21	19.5	1.5	92
FRUIT JUICES AND PUNCHES					
Acerola cherry juice unsweetened	1 cup	12	11	1	56
Apple raspberry cherry juice cocktail, ready-to-drink	1 cup	33	33	na	130

FRUITS AND FRUIT JUICES

FOOD	SERVING	TOTAL CARBS (G)	NET CARBS (G)	FIBER (G)	CALORIES
Apple juice, canned or bottled	1 cup	29	29	t	117
Apple juice, from concentrate	1 cup	28	28	t	112
Apricot nectar, canned	1 cup	36	34.5	1.5	141
Cranberry-apple juice drink, bottled	1 cup	42	42	t	164
Cranberry-apricot juice drink, bottled	1 cup	40	40	t	157
Cranberry-grape juice drink, bottled	1 cup	34	34	t	137
Cranberry juice cocktail, bottled	1 cup	36	36	t	144
Cranberry juice cocktail, frozen concentrate, prepared w/water	1 cup	35	35	t	138
Cranberry juice, cocktail, low calorie	1 cup	11	11	0	45
Fruit punch drink, canned	1 cup	30	30	t	117
Fruit punch drink, frozen concentrate, prepared w/water	1 cup	29	29	t	114
Fruit punch, ready-to-drink	1 serving	26	26	0	99
Fruit punch–flavor drink, powder, w/added sodium, prepared w/water	1 cup	25	25	0	97

FRUITS AND FRUIT JUICES 247

FOOD	SERVING	TOTAL CARBS (G)	NET CARBS (G)	FIBER (G)	CALORIES
Fruit punch–flavor drink, powder, w/o added sodium, prepared w/water	1 cup	25	25	0	97
Grape berry punch, ready-to-drink	1 serving	31	31	0	116
Grape juice, canned or bottled	1 cup	38	38	t	154
Grape juice drink, canned	1 cup	32	32	t	125
Grapefruit juice, canned	1 cup	22	22	t	94
Grapefruit juice, from concentrate	1 cup	24	24	t	101
Grapefruit juice, pink, fresh	1 cup	23	23	na	96
Grapefruit juice, white, fresh	1 cup	23	23	t	96
Lemonade mix, w/vitamin C	1 portion, ⅛ cap/tub	18	18	na	64
Lemonade, pink, frozen concentrate, prepared w/water	1 cup	26	26	0	99
Lemonade, powder, prepared w/water	1 cup	27	27	0	103
Lemonade, white, frozen concentrate, prepared w/water	1 cup	26	26	t	99
Lemonade-flavor drink, powder, prepared w/water	1 cup	29	29	0	112

FRUITS AND FRUIT JUICES

FOOD	SERVING	TOTAL CARBS (G)	NET CARBS (G)	FIBER (G)	CALORIES
Lemon juice, bottled	1 tbsp	1	1	0	3
Lemon juice, raw	yield from 1 lemon	4	4	0	12
Lime juice, raw	yield from 1 lime	3	3	0	10
Orange juice, California, from concentrate	1 cup	25	25	na	110
Orange & apricot juice drink, canned	1 cup	32	32	t	128
Orange juice, canned	1 cup	25	20	.5	105
Orange juice, from concentrate	1 cup	25	20	.5	110
Orange juice, fresh	1 cup	26	25.5	.5	112
Orange-grapefruit, canned	1 cup	25	25	t	106
Papaya nectar, canned	1 cup	36	34.5	1.5	143
Peach nectar, canned	1 cup	35	33.5	1.5	134
Pear nectar, canned	1 cup	39	37.5	1.5	150
Passion-fruit juice, purple, fresh	1 cup	34	33.5	.5	126
Passion-fruit juice, yellow, fresh	1 cup	36	35.5	.5	148
Pineapple & grapefruit juice drink, canned	1 cup	29	29	t	118
Pineapple juice, canned	1 cup	34	33.5	.5	140
Pineapple juice, from concentrate	1 cup	32	31.5	.5	130
Pineapple & orange juice drink, canned	1 cup	30	30	t	125
Prune juice, canned	½ cup	22	21	1	91
Sports drink, lemon lime flavor mix, powder	¾ scoop	15	15	0	58

FOOD	SERVING	TOTAL CARBS (G)	NET CARBS (G)	FIBER (G)	CALORIES
Tangerine juice, fresh	1 cup	25	24.5	.5	106
Tropical punch, ready-to-drink	1 serving	24	24	0	90
Tropical punch, powder, prepared w/water	1 serving	16	16	0	64

GAME MEATS, LEAN

FOOD	SERVING	TOTAL CARBS (G)	NET CARBS (G)	FIBER (G)	CALORIES
Bison, chuck roast, lean only, braised	4 oz	0	0	0	218
Bison, ribeye, lean only	4 oz	0	0	0	131
Bison, lean only, roasted	4 oz	0	0	0	162
Bison, top round, lean only, broiled	4 oz	0	0	0	197
Bison, top sirloin, lean only, broiled	4 oz	0	0	0	193
Rabbit, domesticated, various cuts, roasted	4 oz	0	0	0	223
Rabbit, domesticated, various cuts, stewed	4 oz	0	0	0	233
Rabbit, wild, various cuts, stewed	4 oz	0	0	0	196
Venison, ground, pan-broiled	4 oz	0	0	0	211
Venison, loin, lean only, broiled	4 oz	0	0	0	170
Venison, roasted	4 oz	0	0	0	179
Venison, shoulder roast, lean only, braised	4 oz	0	0	0	216
Venison, tenderloin, lean only, broiled	4 oz	0	0	0	168

250 GRAINS AND GRAIN CAKES

FOOD	SERVING	TOTAL CARBS (G)	NET CARBS (G)	FIBER (G)	CALORIES
Venison, top round, lean only, broiled	4 oz	0	0	0	172

GRAINS AND GRAIN CAKES
GRAINS

FOOD	SERVING	TOTAL CARBS (G)	NET CARBS (G)	FIBER (G)	CALORIES
Amaranth, dry	¼ cup	32	25	7	182
Barley, pearled, cooked	½ cup	22	19	3	97
Brown rice, long grain, cooked	½ cup	22	20	2	108
Brown rice, medium grain, cooked	½ cup	23	21	2	109
Bulgur, cooked	½ cup	17	13	4	76
Couscous, cooked	½ cup	18	17	1	88
Millet, cooked	½ cup	21	20	1	104
Quinoa, cooked	½ cup	17	15.5	1.5	106
Rice noodles, cooked	½ cup	22	21	1	96
White rice, w/pasta, cooked	½ cup	22	19	3	123
White rice, short grain, cooked	½ cup	27	27	na	121
White rice, medium grain, cooked	½ cup	27	26	t	121
White rice, long grain, cooked	½ cup	22	22	t	103
White rice, long grain, instant, cooked	½ cup	18	17.5	.5	81
White rice, long grain, parboiled, enriched, cooked	½ cup	22	22	t	100

FOOD	SERVING	TOTAL CARBS (G)	NET CARBS (G)	FIBER (G)	CALORIES
GRAIN CAKES					
Brown rice, buckwheat	2 cakes	14	13	1	68
Brown rice, corn	2 cakes	15	14.5	.5	69
Brown rice, multigrain	2 cakes	15	14.5	.5	70
Brown rice, plain	2 cakes	15	14	1	70
Brown rice, rye	2 cakes	15	14	1	69
Brown rice, sesame seed	2 cakes	15	15	na	71
Corn cakes	2 cakes	15	15	t	70
Corn cakes, very low sodium	2 cakes	15	15	na	70
Popcorn cakes	2 cakes	16	15	1	77
HOT DOGS					
Cheesefurter, cheese smoke	1 link	1	1	0	141
Hot dog, beef	1 hot dog	2	2	0	141
Hot dog, beef & pork	1 hot dog	1	1	0	135
Hot dog, fat free	1 serving	2	2	0	37
Hot dog, light pork, turkey, beef	1 serving	2	2	0	111
Hot dog, meat	1 hot dog	2	2	0	151
Hot dog, pork	1 hot dog	t	t	t	204
ICE CREAM AND FROZEN DESSERTS					
ICE CREAM AND SHERBET, GENERIC					
Butter almond	½ cup	14	14	0	167
Butter pecan	½ cup	16	16	0	175
Cherry vanilla	½ cup	16	16	0	144
Chocolate	½ cup	16	16	0	175
Chocolate chip	½ cup	17	17	0	166

252 ICE CREAM AND FROZEN DESSERTS

FOOD	SERVING	TOTAL CARBS (G)	NET CARBS (G)	FIBER (G)	CALORIES
Chocolate/vanilla swirl	½ cup	17	17	0	161
Coffee	½ cup	14	14	0	149
French vanilla	½ cup	19	19	0	185
Neapolitan	½ cup	17	17	0	150
Rocky road	½ cup	21	16	.5	182
Sherbet, orange	½ cup	26	26	0	122
Sherbet, rainbow	½ cup	26	26	0	122
Sorbet	½ cup	30	30	0	120
Strawberry	½ cup	18	18	0	127
Vanilla	½ cup	24	24	0	259
Vanilla, soft serve, ice milk	½ cup	24	24	0	164
Vanilla ice cream w/dark chocolate coating	1 bar	12	12	0	166
ICE CREAM AND SHERBET, BY BRAND					
Atkins Homemade Soft Serve Mix, Chocolate	½ cup	1	1	0	6
Atkins Homemade Soft Serve Mix, Vanilla	½ cup	1	1	0	6
Atkins Endulge Butter Pecan Ice Cream	½ cup	12	3	4	170
Atkins Endulge Chocolate Ice Cream	½ cup	13	3	5	140
Atkins Endulge Chocolate Peanut Butter Swirl Ice Cream	½ cup	14	3	5	179
Atkins Endulge Vanilla Ice Cream	½ cup	13	3	4	140
Atkins Endulge Vanilla Fudge Swirl Ice Cream	½ cup	14	3	4	140

ICE CREAM AND FROZEN DESSERTS 253

FOOD	SERVING	TOTAL CARBS (G)	NET CARBS (G)	FIBER (G)	CALORIES
Ben & Jerry's Carb Karma Ice Cream, Chocolate	½ cup	11	4	5	150
Ben & Jerry's Carb Karma Ice Cream, Half Baked	½ cup	18	5	4	180
Ben & Jerry's Carb Karma Ice Cream, Vanilla Swiss Almond	½ cup	13	2	4	170
Breyers All Natural Light French Vanilla Ice Cream	½ cup	18	18	0	120
Breyers All Natural Light Mint Chocolate Chip Ice Cream	½ cup	20	20	0	130
Breyers All Natural Light Vanilla/Chocolate/Strawberry Ice Cream	½ cup	18	18	0	110
Breyers All Natural Light Vanilla Ice Cream	½ cup	17	17	0	110
Breyers 2% Milk Light Vanilla Ice Cream	½ cup	18	18	0	130
Breyers 98% Fat Free Chocolate Ice Cream	½ cup	21	17	4	90
Breyers 98% Fat Free Vanilla Ice Cream	½ cup	21	17	4	90
Breyers 98% Fat Free No Sugar Added Chocolate Fudge Brownie Ice Cream	½ cup	20	11	4	90
Breyers No Sugar Added Butter Pecan Ice Cream	½ cup	15	11	1	120

254 ICE CREAM AND FROZEN DESSERTS

FOOD	SERVING	TOTAL CARBS (G)	NET CARBS (G)	FIBER (G)	CALORIES
Breyers No Sugar Added Chocolate Caramel Ice Cream	½ cup	18	11	1	110
Breyers No Sugar Added French Vanilla Ice Cream	½ cup	14	11	0	110
Breyers No Sugar Added Vanilla Fudge Twirl Ice Cream	½ cup	19	11	1	110
Breyers No Sugar Added Vanilla/ Chocolate/Strawberry Ice Cream	½ cup	15	12	0	100
Breyers No Sugar Added Vanilla Ice Cream	½ cup	15	12	0	100
Breyers No Sugar Added Vanilla/ Chocolate/Strawberry Ice Cream	½ cup	15	12	0	100
Breyers No Sugar Added Vanilla Ice Cream	½ cup	15	12	0	100
Breyers Carb Smart Butter Pecan Ice Cream	½ cup	10	4	3	150
Breyers Carb Smart Chocolate Almond Ice Cream	½ cup	10	4	3	150
Breyers Carb Smart Chocolate Ice Cream	½ cup	10	4	3	130
Breyers Carb Smart Mint Chocolate Ice Cream	½ cup	13	4	6	140

ICE CREAM AND FROZEN DESSERTS

FOOD	SERVING	TOTAL CARBS (G)	NET CARBS (G)	FIBER (G)	CALORIES
Breyers Carb Smart Rocky Road Ice Cream	½ cup	12	4	3	140
Breyers Carb Smart Strawberry Ice Cream	½ cup	10	4	3	130
Breyers Carb Smart Vanilla Ice Cream	½ cup	10	4	3	130
Keto Ice Cream Mix, Black Raspberry, Prepared w/Cream & Skim Milk	½ cup	7	4	6	170
Keto Ice Cream Mix, Chocolate, Prepared w/Cream & Skim Milk	½ cup	7	4	6	170
Keto Ice Cream Mix, Orange & Crème, Prepared w/Cream & Skim Milk	½ cup	6	4	6	170
Keto Ice Cream Mix, Strawberry, Prepared w/Cream & Skim Milk	½ cup	7	4	6	170
Keto Sherbet Mix, Orange, Prepared w/Skim Milk	½ cup	8	2	.5	174
FROZEN AND CHILLED DESSERTS, BY BRAND					
Atkins Mousse Mix	1 tbsp	4	0	4	24
Expert Foods Wise CHOice Mousse Mix	1 tbsp	4	0	4	240

256 ICE CREAM BARS AND POPS

FOOD	SERVING	TOTAL CARBS (G)	NET CARBS (G)	FIBER (G)	CALORIES
Expert Foods Wise CHOice Frozen Dessert Mix	⅛ package	4	0	4	24

ICE CREAM BARS AND POPS
ICE CREAM BARS, BY BRAND

FOOD	SERVING	TOTAL CARBS (G)	NET CARBS (G)	FIBER (G)	CALORIES
Atkins Frozen Fudge Bar Mix	2 bars	4	1.3	4	22
Atkins Endulge Ice Cream Bars, Chocolate Fudge	1 bar	12	2	5	130
Atkins Endulge Ice Cream Bars, Chocolate Fudge Swirl	1 bar	12	3	4	180
Atkins Endulge Ice Cream Bars, Peanut Butter Swirl	1 bar	12	2	4	180
Atkins Endulge Ice Cream Bars, Vanilla Fudge Swirl	1 bar	12	3	4	180
Breyers No Sugar Added Fruit Bars	1 bar (1.75 fl oz)	5	3	0	25
Expert Foods Wise CHOice Frozen Fudge Bar mix	⅑ pkg (6 g)	4	0	4	95
Silhouette Brands Skinny Carb Bar, Chocolate Peanut Butter	1 bar	13	3	5	150

FOOD	SERVING	TOTAL CARBS (G)	NET CARBS (G)	FIBER (G)	CALORIES
Silhouette Brands Skinny Carb Bar, Vanilla Caramel Pecan	1 bar	14	3	5	140
ICE CREAM BARS					
Fruit bar	1 bar	11	11	0	44
Fudgesicle	1 bar	9	9	na	45
Ice cream sandwich	1 bar	21	21	0	159
ICE CREAM SANDWICHES, BY BRAND					
Silhouette Brands Skinny Carb Light Ice Cream Sandwich, Chocolate	1 sandwich	21	7	7	140
Silhouette Brands Skinny Carb Light Ice Cream Sandwich, Vanilla	1 sandwich	21	7	7	140

JAM, SUGAR, SYRUP, AND SWEETENERS

HONEY, JAMS, PRESERVES, AND JELLIES, GENERIC

FOOD	SERVING	TOTAL CARBS (G)	NET CARBS (G)	FIBER (G)	CALORIES
Apple butter	1 tbsp	7	7	t	29
Honey, strained or extracted	1 tbsp	17	17	0	64
Jams & preserves	1 tbsp	14	14	t	56
Jams & preserves	1 pkt	10	10	t	39
Jam, apricot	1 tbsp	13	13	t	48
Jam, apricot	1 pkt	9	9	t	34
Jam, strawberry	1 tbsp	14	14	0	60
Jellies, all types	1 tbsp	13	13	t	54
Jellies, all types	1 pkt	10	10	t	40
Jelly, grape	1 tbsp	14	14	0	50

258 JAM, SUGAR, SYRUP, AND SWEETENERS

FOOD	SERVING	TOTAL CARBS (G)	NET CARBS (G)	FIBER (G)	CALORIES
Orange marmalade	1 tbsp	13	13	0	49
Orange marmalade	1 pkt	9	9	0	34
Strawberry spread, all fruit	1 tbsp	10	10	na	42
HONEY, JAMS, PRESERVES, AND JELLIES, BY BRAND, LOW CARB					
Steel's Apricot Jam	1 tbsp (18 g)	2	2	0	9
Steel's Champagne Peach Jam	1 tbsp (18 g)	1.5	1.5	0	6
Steel's Gourmet Jam	1 tbsp (18 g)	2	2	0	9
Steel's Red Raspberry Jam	1 tbsp (18 g)	1	1	0	10
Steel's Sour Cherry Jam	1 tbsp (18 g)	1.5	1.5	0	6
Steel's Strawberry Jam	1 tbsp (18 g)	1.5	1.5	0	6
Steel's Wild Blueberry Jam	1 tbsp (18 g)	2.3	2.3	0	9
SUGARS					
Brown	3 tsp unpacked	9	9	0	34
Maple	3 tsp	8	8	0	32
Powdered	3 tsp	7	7	0	29
White	1 lump (2 cubes)	5	5	0	19
White	1 pkt	6	6	0	23
White	3 tsp	13	13	0	49
SWEETENERS AND SUGAR SUBSTITUTES, BY BRAND					
DiabetiSweet Brown Sugar Substitute	1 tsp	4.3	.1	0	10
DiabetiSweet Sugar Substitute	1 tsp	4.4	0	0	8.9
Dixie Diners' Club "Not-Sugar" Sugar Substitute	⅕ tsp	t	t	0	0

JAM, SUGAR, SYRUP, AND SWEETENERS

FOOD	SERVING	TOTAL CARBS (G)	NET CARBS (G)	FIBER (G)	CALORIES
Fran Gare's Xylitol Miracle Sweet	1 tsp	1	1	0	9.6
Low Carb Success Erythritol	1 tbsp	15	0	0	3
Perfect Sweet Xylitol	1 tsp	1	1	0	9.6
Steel's Maltitol Brown Nature Sweet Crystals	1 tsp	3	0	0	6
Steel's Maltitol Nature Sweet Crystals	1 tsp	4	0	0	8
Steel's Maltitol Nature Sweet Honey Flavor	1 tsp	6	0	0	24
Steel's Maltitol Nature Sweet Vanilla Flavor	1 tsp	6	0	0	24
Steel's Maltitol Powdered Nature Sweet	1 tsp	3	0	0	6
Stevita Organic Stevia, in Packets	1 pkt	0	0	0	0
Stevita Organic Stevia, Spoonable	1/3 tsp	0	0	0	0
Stevita Stevia, Liquid	1/8 tsp	0	0	0	0
Stevita Stevia Supreme, Spoonable	1/3 tsp	0	0	0	0
Stevita Stevia Supreme, in Packets	1 pkt	0	0	0	0
Stevita Ultimate Stevia, Pure Stevia Extract, Spoonable	1/32 tsp	0	0	0	0

JAM, SUGAR, SYRUP, AND SWEETENERS

FOOD	SERVING	TOTAL CARBS (G)	NET CARBS (G)	FIBER (G)	CALORIES
SYRUPS, BY BRAND					
Atkins Quick Quisine Sugar Free Cherry Syrup	1 tbsp	0	0	0	0
Atkins Quick Quisine Sugar Free Chocolate Syrup	1 tbsp	0	0	0	0
Atkins Quick Quisine Sugar Free Hazelnut Syrup	1 tbsp	0	0	0	0
Atkins Quick Quisine Sugar Free Pancake Syrup	2 oz	0	0	0	0
Atkins Quick Quisine Sugar Free Raspberry Syrup	1 tbsp	0	0	0	0
Atkins Quick Quisine Sugar Free Strawberry Syrup	1 tbsp	0	0	0	0
Atkins Quick Quisine Sugar Free Vanilla Syrup	1 tbsp	0	0	0	0
Atkins Quick Quisine Sugar Free Soda Flavored Syrup, Cola	1 tbsp	0	0	0	0
Atkins Quick Quisine Sugar Free Soda Flavored Syrup, Ginger Ale	1 tbsp	0	0	0	0

JAM, SUGAR, SYRUP, AND SWEETENERS

FOOD	SERVING	TOTAL CARBS (G)	NET CARBS (G)	FIBER (G)	CALORIES
Atkins Quick Quisine Sugar Free Soda Flavored Syrup, Lemon-Lime	1 tbsp	0	0	0	0
Atkins Quick Quisine Sugar Free Soda Flavored Syrup, Root Beer	1 tbsp	0	0	0	0
Da Vinci Gourmet Sugar Free Almond Syrup	1 tbsp	0	0	0	0
Da Vinci Gourmet Sugar Free Amaretto Syrup	1 tbsp	0	0	0	0
Da Vinci Gourmet Sugar Free B-52 Syrup	1 tbsp	0	0	0	0
Da Vinci Gourmet Sugar Free Banana Syrup	1 tbsp	0	0	0	0
Da Vinci Gourmet Sugar Free Blueberry Syrup	1 tbsp	0	0	0	0
Da Vinci Gourmet Sugar Free Butter Rum Syrup	1 tbsp	0	0	0	0
Da Vinci Gourmet Sugar Free Caramel Syrup	1 tbsp	0	0	0	0
Da Vinci Gourmet Sugar Free Cherry Syrup	1 tbsp	0	0	0	0

JAM, SUGAR, SYRUP, AND SWEETENERS

FOOD	SERVING	TOTAL CARBS (G)	NET CARBS (G)	FIBER (G)	CALORIES
Da Vinci Gourmet Sugar Free Chocolate Syrup	1 tbsp	0	0	0	0
Da Vinci Gourmet Sugar Free Cinnamon Syrup	1 tbsp	0	0	0	0
Da Vinci Gourmet Sugar Free Coconut Syrup	1 tbsp	0	0	0	0
Da Vinci Gourmet Sugar Free Cola Syrup	1 tbsp	0	0	0	0
Da Vinci Gourmet Sugar Free Cookie Dough Syrup	1 tbsp	0	0	0	0
Da Vinci Gourmet Sugar Free Crème de Menthe Syrup	1 tbsp	0	0	0	0
Da Vinci Gourmet Sugar Free Danish Pastry Syrup	1 tbsp	0	0	0	0
Da Vinci Gourmet Sugar Free Dulce de Leche Syrup	1 tbsp	0	0	0	0
Da Vinci Gourmet Sugar Free Egg Nog Syrup	1 tbsp	0	0	0	0
Da Vinci Gourmet Sugar Free English Toffee Syrup	1 tbsp	0	0	0	0

JAM, SUGAR, SYRUP, AND SWEETENERS

FOOD	SERVING	TOTAL CARBS (G)	NET CARBS (G)	FIBER (G)	CALORIES
Da Vinci Gourmet Sugar Free French Vanilla Syrup	1 tbsp	0	0	0	0
Da Vinci Gourmet Sugar Free German Chocolate Cake Syrup	1 tbsp	0	0	0	0
Da Vinci Gourmet Sugar Free Grape Syrup	1 tbsp	0	0	0	0
Da Vinci Gourmet Sugar Free Green Apple Syrup	1 tbsp	0	0	0	0
Da Vinci Gourmet Sugar Free Hazelnut Syrup	1 tbsp	0	0	0	0
Da Vinci Gourmet Sugar Free Huckleberry Syrup	1 tbsp	0	0	0	0
Da Vinci Gourmet Sugar Free Irish Cream Syrup	1 tbsp	0	0	0	0
Da Vinci Gourmet Sugar Free Kahlúa Syrup	1 tbsp	0	0	0	0
Da Vinci Gourmet Sugar Free Macadamia Syrup	1 tbsp	0	0	0	0
Da Vinci Gourmet Sugar Free Orange Syrup	1 tbsp	0	0	0	0

JAM, SUGAR, SYRUP, AND SWEETENERS

FOOD	SERVING	TOTAL CARBS (G)	NET CARBS (G)	FIBER (G)	CALORIES
Da Vinci Gourmet Sugar Free Pancake Syrup	1 tbsp	0	0	0	0
Da Vinci Gourmet Sugar Free Peach Syrup	1 tbsp	0	0	0	0
Da Vinci Gourmet Sugar Free Peanut Butter Syrup	1 tbsp	0	0	0	0
Da Vinci Gourmet Sugar Free Peppermint Paddy Syrup	1 tbsp	0	0	0	0
Da Vinci Gourmet Sugar Free Pineapple Syrup	1 tbsp	0	0	0	0
Da Vinci Gourmet Sugar Free Raspberry Syrup	1 tbsp	0	0	0	0
Da Vinci Gourmet Sugar Free Root Beer Syrup	1 tbsp	0	0	0	0
Da Vinci Gourmet Sugar Free Spice Blend Syrup	1 tbsp	0	0	0	0
Da Vinci Gourmet Sugar Free Strawberry Syrup	1 tbsp	0	0	0	0
Da Vinci Gourmet Sugar Free Toasted Marshmallow Syrup	1 tbsp	0	0	0	0

JAM, SUGAR, SYRUP, AND SWEETENERS

FOOD	SERVING	TOTAL CARBS (G)	NET CARBS (G)	FIBER (G)	CALORIES
Da Vinci Gourmet Sugar Free Vanilla Syrup	1 tbsp	0	0	0	0
Da Vinci Gourmet Sugar Free Watermelon Syrup	1 tbsp	0	0	0	0
Da Vinci Gourmet Sugar Free White Chocolate Syrup	1 tbsp	0	0	0	0
Joseph's Sugar Free Syrup, Maple Flavor	¼ cup	9	0	0	35
Keto Syrup, Maple/Butter Flavor	¼ cup	1	1	0	4
Ketogenics Zero-Carb Pancake Syrup	¼ cup	1	0	1	4
Steel's Chocolate Flavor Syrup	2 tbsp	12	4	0	50
Steel's Country Raspberry Syrup	2 tbsp	9	0	1	36
Steel's Country Syrup, Real Maple Flavor	2 tbsp	16	0	0	64
Steel's Wild Blueberry Syrup	2 tbsp	10	1	0	30
Walden Farms Chocolate Flavored Syrup	2 tbsp	0	0	0	0
Walden Farms Pancake Syrup, Maple Flavor	¼ cup	0	0	0	0

FOOD	SERVING	TOTAL CARBS (G)	NET CARBS (G)	FIBER (G)	CALORIES
SYRUPS, GENERIC					
Blends, cane & 15% maple	1 tbsp	15	15	0	56
Blends, corn, refiner & sugar	1 tbsp	17	17	0	64
Chocolate syrup, fudge type	2 tbsp	24	23	1	133
Corn, dark	1 tbsp	15	15	0	56
Corn, high fructose	1 tbsp	14	14	0	53
Corn, light	1 tbsp	15	15	0	56
Fruit syrup	1 tbsp	14	14	0	53
Malt	1 tbsp	17	17	0	76
Maple syrup	1 tbsp	13	13	0	52
Molasses	1 tbsp	15	15	0	58
Pancake, regular	1 tbsp	15	15	0	57
Pancake, w/butter	1 tbsp	15	15	0	59
Pancake, w/2% maple	1 tbsp	14	14	0	53
Sorghum	1 tbsp	15	15	0	61
LAMB					
Lamb, ground, broiled	4 oz	0	0	0	320
Leg, shank half, lean only, trimmed to ¼" fat, choice, roasted	4 oz	0	0	0	204
Leg, shank half, lean & fat, trimmed to ¼" fat, choice, roasted	4 oz	0	0	0	246
Leg, sirloin half, lean only, trimmed to ¼" fat, choice, roasted	4 oz	0	0	0	231

FOOD	SERVING	TOTAL CARBS (G)	NET CARBS (G)	FIBER (G)	CALORIES
Leg, whole (shank & sirloin), lean only, trimmed to ¼" fat, choice, roasted	4 oz	0	0	0	216
Loin, lean only, trimmed to ¼" fat, choice, broiled	4 oz	0	0	0	245
Loin, lean only, trimmed to ¼" fat, choice, roasted	4 oz	0	0	0	229
Retail cuts, lean & fat, trimmed to ⅛" fat, choice, cooked	4 oz	0	0	0	307
Rib, lean & fat, trimmed to ⅛" fat, choice, broiled	4 oz	0	0	0	385
Rib, lean & fat, trimmed to ⅛" fat, choice, roasted	4 oz	0	0	0	386
Rib, lean & fat, trimmed to ¼" fat, choice, broiled	4 oz	0	0	0	409
Rib, lean & fat, trimmed to ¼" fat, choice, roasted	4 oz	0	0	0	407
Shoulder/arm, lean only, trimmed to ¼" fat, choice, broiled	4 oz	0	0	0	227
Shoulder/arm, lean only, trimmed to ¼" fat, choice, roasted	4 oz	0	0	0	218

FOOD	SERVING	TOTAL CARBS (G)	NET CARBS (G)	FIBER (G)	CALORIES
Shoulder, whole (arm & shoulder), lean only, trimmed to ¼" fat, choice, broiled	4 oz	0	0	0	238
Shoulder, whole (arm & shoulder), lean only, trimmed to ¼" fat, choice, broiled	4 oz	0	0	0	231
Sirloin chop, lean only, broiled	4 oz	0	0	0	213

LUNCH MEATS

FOOD	SERVING	TOTAL CARBS (G)	NET CARBS (G)	FIBER (G)	CALORIES
Beerwurst, beef	1 slice	t	t	0	76
Beerwurst, pork	1 slice	.5	.5	0	55
Blood sausage	1 slice	0	0	0	94
Bologna, beef	1 slice	t	t	0	87
Bologna, beef, Lebanon	1 slice	t	t	0	112
Bologna, fat free	1 serving	2	2	0	22
Bologna, pork	1 slice	t	t	0	69
Bologna, pork & beef	1 slice	1	1	0	87
Bologna, pork & turkey, lite	2 slices	2	2	0	118
Bologna, turkey	2 slices	t	t	0	113
Bratwurst, beef & pork, smoked	2 oz	1.5	1.5	0	168
Bratwurst, veal, cooked	2 oz	0	0	0	194
Braunschweiger	1 slice	.5	.5	0	65
Chicken, smoked	2 oz	t	t	0	94
Chicken, White, Oven Roasted (Louis Rich)	1 serving	1	1	0	36

LUNCH MEATS

FOOD	SERVING	TOTAL CARBS (G)	NET CARBS (G)	FIBER (G)	CALORIES
Chicken, White, Oven Roasted Deluxe (Louis Rich)	1 serving	1	1	0	28
Chicken Breast Classic Baked (Louis Rich)	2 slices	2	2	0	43
Chicken Breast, Honey Glazed (Oscar Mayer)	2 slices	1	1	0	28
Chicken breast, oven roasted, fat free	2 slices	1	1	0	33
Chicken breast, smoked, mesquite flavor	2 slices	1	1	0	34
Ham, extra lean	2 slices	t	t	0	73
Ham, 96% Fat Free (Oscar Mayer)	2 slices	1	1	0	44
Liverwurst	1 slice	t	t	0	59
Pastrami, beef, 98% fat free	6 slices	1	1	0	54
Salami, beef	2 slices	t	t	0	204
Salami, beef & pork	2 slices	1	1	0	115
Salami, turkey	2 slices	t	t	0	82
Summer sausage, w/cheese	2 oz	1	1	t	242
Swisswurst, pork & beef, w/Swiss cheese, smoked	1 serving (2.7 oz)	1	1	0	236
Turkey Breast, Oven Roasted, Fat Free (Louis Rich)	2 slices	2	2	0	101
Turkey Breast, Smoked (Oscar Mayer)	2 slices	1	1	0	21

FOOD	SERVING	TOTAL CARBS (G)	NET CARBS (G)	FIBER (G)	CALORIES
Turkey Breast & White Turkey, Smoked (Louis Rich)	2 slices	1	1	0	56
Turkey ham	2 slices	t	t	0	64
Turkey ham, cured turkey thigh meat	2 slices	t	t	0	73

MILK AND MILK BEVERAGES

FOOD	SERVING	TOTAL CARBS (G)	NET CARBS (G)	FIBER (G)	CALORIES
Buttermilk, low fat	1 cup	12	12	0	98
Chocolate milk	1 cup	26	24	2	208
Chocolate-flavored beverage mix, prepared w/whole milk	1 cup	31	30	1	226
Chocolate syrup, prepared w/whole milk	1 cup	36	35	1	257
Cocoa, sugar-free mix, mixed w/water	1 pkt	11	10	1	54
Coconut milk, canned	1 cup	6	6	na	445
Dairy Beverage, Carb Countdown, Fat Free (Hood)	1 cup	3	3	0	70
Dairy Beverage, Carb Countdown, Homogenized (Hood)	1 cup	3	3	0	130
Dairy Beverage, Carb Countdown, 2% (Hood)	1 cup	3	3	3	120

MILK AND MILK BEVERAGES

FOOD	SERVING	TOTAL CARBS (G)	NET CARBS (G)	FIBER (G)	CALORIES
Dairy Beverage, Carb Countdown, 2% Chocolate (Hood)	1 cup	3	2	1	100
Dry milk, nonfat, instant	⅓ cup	12	12	0	82
Eggnog	1 cup	34	34	0	343
Eggnog-flavored mix, prepared w/whole milk	1 cup	39	38	1	261
Evaporated milk, canned, nonfat	½ cup	15	15	0	100
Hot cocoa, homemade	1 cup	29	27	2	193
Hot Cocoa Mix (Atkins)	3 tbsp	3	3	0	50
Hot Cocoa in Packets (Keto)	1 pkt (10 g)	6	2	4	40
Low-fat milk, 1%, protein fortified	1 cup	14	14	0	118
Low-fat milk, 1%, regular	1 cup	12	12	0	102
Malted drink mix, prepared w/whole milk	1 cup	30	30	t	236
Milk, canned, condensed, sweetened	½ cup	83	83	0	491
Milk shake, chocolate	8 fl oz	48	47	1	270
Milk shake, vanilla	8 fl oz	40	40	0	254
Milk substitutes, fluid, w/hydrogenated vegetable oils	1 cup	15	15	0	149
Nonfat milk (skim or fat free)	1 cup	12	12	0	86
Reduced-fat milk, 2%	1 cup	12	12	0	122

NUTRITIONAL DRINKS AND SHAKES

FOOD	SERVING	TOTAL CARBS (G)	NET CARBS (G)	FIBER (G)	CALORIES
Strawberry-flavored beverage mix, prepared w/whole milk	1 cup	33	33	0	234
Whole milk	1 cup	11	11	0	156
NUTRITIONAL DRINKS AND SHAKES					
Atkins Morning Start Drink Mix, Apple	8 fl oz	0	0	0	0
Atkins Morning Start Drink Mix, Fruit Punch	8 fl oz	0	0	0	0
Atkins Morning Start Drink Mix, Orange	8 fl oz	0	0	0	0
Atkins Morning Start Drink Mix, Peach Iced Tea	8 fl oz	0	0	0	0
Atkins Ready-To-Drink Shakes, Café au Lait	1 can (11 oz)	5	2	3	170
Atkins Ready-To-Drink Shakes, Chocolate Delight	1 can (11 oz)	6	1	3	170
Atkins Ready-To-Drink Shakes, Chocolate Royale	1 can (11 oz)	6	2	4	170
Atkins Ready-To-Drink Shakes, Strawberry	1 can (11 oz)	4	2	2	170
Atkins Ready-To-Drink Shakes, Vanilla	1 can (11 oz)	4	1	3	170
Atkins Shake Mix, Cappuccino	2 scoops	10	3	5	140

NUTRITIONAL DRINKS AND SHAKES 273

FOOD	SERVING	TOTAL CARBS (G)	NET CARBS (G)	FIBER (G)	CALORIES
Atkins Shake Mix, Chocolate	2 scoops	10	3	5	140
Atkins Shake Mix, Strawberry	2 scoops	9	3	4	130
Atkins Shake Mix, Vanilla	2 scoops	9	3	4	130
Atkins Electrolyte Refresher Sports Drink, Fruit Punch	1 serving (8 fl oz)	0	0	0	0
Atkins Electrolyte Refresher Sports Drink, Lemon-Lime	1 serving (8 fl oz)	0	0	0	0
Atkins Electrolyte Refresher Sports Drink, Orange	1 serving (8 fl oz)	0	0	0	0
Boost, regular	1 can (8 fl oz)	41	41	0	240
Boost, high protein	1 can (8 fl oz)	33	33	0	255
Carb Options Chocolate Delight Shake	1 can	6	2	4	190
Carb Options Creamy Vanilla Shake	1 can	6	2	4	190
CarboRite Ready to Drink Shake, Creamy Vanilla	1 can (325 ml)	7	1	2	170
CarboRite Ready to Drink Shake, Rich Chocolate	1 can (325 ml)	10	2	3	170
CarboRite Shake Mix, Banana Blitz	2 scoops (38 g)	8	3	5	150
CarboRite Shake Mix, Chocolate Supreme	2 scoops (42 g)	8	3	5	150

NUTRITIONAL DRINKS AND SHAKES

FOOD	SERVING	TOTAL CARBS (G)	NET CARBS (G)	FIBER (G)	CALORIES
CarboRite Shake Mix, Strawberry Crème	2 scoops (38 g)	8	3	5	150
CarboRite Shake Mix, Vanilla	2 scoops (42 g)	8	3	5	150
DiebetiTrim Nutrition Drink Mix, Chocolate	1 pkt (28.6 g)	10	6	4	90
DiebetiTrim Nutrition Drink Mix, Vanilla	1 pkt (28.6 g)	10	6	4	90
Doctor's CarbRite Diet Smoothie Mix, Smooth Vanilla	1 scoop (30 g)	2	2	0	114
Emer'gen-C Lite Energy Booster, Light Natural Citrus Flavor	1 pkt (4 g)	.13	.13	0	1
Ensure, regular	1 can (8 fl oz)	40	40	0	250
Ensure Fiber w/FOS	1 can (8 fl oz)	42	39	3	360
Ensure Plus, high protein	1 can (8 fl oz)	50	50	0	350
Equate Plus, Strawberry, Vanilla & Chocolate	1 can (8 fl oz)	50	50	0	350
Equate Weight Loss Shake, Strawberries & Cream	1 can (11 fl oz)	47	47	na	370
Fruit juice mixable formula, powdered, not reconstituted	1 scoop	17	11	6	240
GeniSoy Shake, vanilla	1 scoop, dry (1.2 oz)	18	18	0	210
Keto High Fiber Complex Powder, Sugar Free, Apple Berry Flavor	1 heaping tsp (8.8 g) per 8 oz liquid	5	2	5	20

NUTRITIONAL DRINKS AND SHAKES 275

FOOD	SERVING	TOTAL CARBS (G)	NET CARBS (G)	FIBER (G)	CALORIES
Keto RTD Chocolate Shake	1 container (11 fl oz)	4	2	2	170
Keto RTD Orange Crème Shake	1 container (11 fl oz)	3	1	2	170
Keto RTD Strawberry Shake	1 container (11 fl oz)	3	1	2	170
Keto RTD Vanilla Shake	1 container (11 fl oz)	3	1	2	170
Keto Shake Banana Crème Mix	2 scoops (44 g)	8	1	7	210
Keto Shake Cappuccino Mix	2 scoops (45 g)	8	1	7	210
Keto Shake Chocolate Mix	2 scoops (45.5 g)	9	2	7	210
Keto Shake Chocolate Peanut Butter Mix	2 scoops (45 g)	9	2	7	210
Keto Shake Eggnog Mix	2 scoops (45 g)	8	1	7	210
Keto Shake Orange Crème Mix	2 scoops (45 g)	8	1	7	210
Keto Shake Strawberry Mix	2 scoops (45 g)	8	1	7	210
Keto Shake Peaches & Crème Mix	2 scoops (45 g)	8	1	7	210
Keto Shake Vanilla Mix	2 scoops (44.5 g)	8	1	7	210
Keto Soy Shake Banana Mix	2 scoops (41 g)	5	3	2	190
Keto Soy Shake Chocolate Fudge Mix	2 scoops (41 g)	5	3	2	190
Keto Soy Shake French Vanilla Mix	2 scoops (41 g)	5	3	2	190

NUTRITIONAL DRINKS AND SHAKES

FOOD	SERVING	TOTAL CARBS (G)	NET CARBS (G)	FIBER (G)	CALORIES
Keto Soy Shake Strawberry Mix	2 scoops (41 g)	5	3	2	190
Labrada CarbWatchers Lean Body Shake Mix, Banana Crème	1 pkt (62 g)	12	11	1	230
Labrada CarbWatchers Lean Body Shake Mix, Dutch Chocolate Ice Cream	1 pkt (62 g)	12	11	1	230
Labrada CarbWatchers Lean Body Shake Mix, Soft Vanilla Ice Cream	1 pkt (62 g)	12	11	1	230
Labrada CarbWatchers Lean Body Shake Mix, Wild Strawberry	1 pkt (62 g)	12	11	1	230
Milk-based liquid, high protein	1 cup	33	33	0	162
Met-Rx Drink Mix, Original	1 serving, pkt (2.5 oz)	19	19	0	250
Myoplex CarbSense Ready to Drink Shake, Chocolate Fudge	11 fl oz	5	3	2	150
Myoplex CarbSense Ready to Drink Shake, French Vanilla	11 fl oz	5	3	2	150
Myoplex CarbSense Ready to Drink Shake, Strawberry Cream	11 fl oz	5	3	2	150

NUTRITIONAL DRINKS AND SHAKES 277

FOOD	SERVING	TOTAL CARBS (G)	NET CARBS (G)	FIBER (G)	CALORIES
Positrim Drink Mix, not reconstituted (Amway Nutrilite)	1 pkt	27	27	0	220
Promax Drink mix (SportPharma)	1 serving (2 scoops)	6	6	0	251
Reduced-calorie meal replacement shake, generic	1 can	38	34	4	250
RxFuel Shake (TwinLab)	1 serving	62	62	na	128
Shake, isotonic liquid nutrition w/fiber (Jevity)	237 ml	37	34	3	261
Shake, isotonic liquid nutrition (Jevity)	1 can (8 fl oz)	36	36	na	250
Slim Fast Ready To Drink Shake, Creamy Chocolate	1 can	8	2	6	190
Slim Fast Ready To Drink Shake, Creamy Vanilla	1 can	7	2	5	190
Stevita Delight Chocolate Flavor Drink Mix	2 tsp (3.3 g)	2	1.5	.5	13
Stevita Bright, Orange Flavor Drink Mix	1 tsp (4 g)	0	0	0	0
Stevita Fresh, Lime Flavor Drink Mix	1 tsp (4 g)	0	0	0	0
Stevita Spring, Grape Flavor Drink Mix	1 tsp (4 g)	0	0	0	0
Stevita Tropical, Orange Flavor Drink Mix	1 tsp (4 g)	0	0	0	0

NUTS, NUT BUTTERS, AND SEEDS

NUTS AND SEEDS, GENERIC

FOOD	SERVING	TOTAL CARBS (G)	NET CARBS (G)	FIBER (G)	CALORIES
Almonds, dry roasted	1 tbsp	2	1	1	51
Almonds, honey roasted	1 tbsp	2.5	1.5	1	53
Almonds, oil roasted	1 tbsp	2	1	1	60
Brazil nuts, dried	1 tbsp	1	.5	.5	57
Cashews, dry roasted	1 tbsp	3	3	t	49
Cashews, oil roasted	1 tbsp	2	2	t	47
Coconut meat, dried, not sweetened	1 tbsp	3	1	2	94
Coconut meat, dried, sweetened, flaked, canned	½ cup	16	14	2	171
Coconut meat, dried, sweetened, flaked, packaged	½ cup	18	16	2	175
Coconut meat, dried, sweetened, shredded	½ cup	22	20	2	233
Hazelnuts or filberts	1 tbsp	1	0	1	53
Hickory nuts, dried	1 tbsp	1	.5	.5	49
Macadamia nuts, dry roasted	1 tbsp	1	0	1	60
Mixed nuts, dry roasted	1 tbsp	2	1	1	51
Mixed nuts, oil roasted, w/peanuts	1 tbsp	2	1	1	55
Mixed nuts, oil roasted, w/o peanuts	1 tbsp	2	1.5	.5	55
Peanuts,* all types, boiled	½ cup	19	11	8	286

* Although peanuts are technically a legume, most people think of them as nuts.

NUTS, NUT BUTTERS, AND SEEDS

FOOD	SERVING	TOTAL CARBS (G)	NET CARBS (G)	FIBER (G)	CALORIES
Peanuts,* all types, dry roasted	10 peanuts	2	1	1	59
Peanuts, oil roasted	1 tbsp	2	1	1	51
Pecans	1 tbsp	1	0	1	47
Pecans, oil roasted	1 tbsp	1	0	1	49
Pistachio nuts, dry roasted	1 tbsp	2	1	1	45
Sunflower seeds, dried	1 tbsp	2	1	1	57
Sunflower seeds, dry roasted	1 tbsp	2	1	1	52
Sunflower seeds, oil roasted	1 tbsp	1	0	1	58
Sunflower seeds, toasted	1 tbsp	2	1	1	58
Trail mix, tropical	1 cup	92	92	0	570
Trail mix, regular, w/chocolate chips, nuts & seeds	1 cup	66	66	0	707
Walnuts, English	1 tbsp	1	0	t	41
NUTS AND SEEDS, BY BRAND					
Atkins Chocolate Almonds	11 pieces	18	2	3	190
Atkins Chocolate Covered Peanuts	25 pieces	18	4	2	190
Atkins Chocolate Covered Macadamias	6 pieces	16	1	2	210
Atkins Chocolate Covered Toffee Bits (Covered Peanuts)	1 bag (8 oz)	24	1	1	170

* Although peanuts are technically a legume, most people think of them as nuts.

NUTS, NUT BUTTERS, AND SEEDS

FOOD	SERVING	TOTAL CARBS (G)	NET CARBS (G)	FIBER (G)	CALORIES
Low Carb Success Sweet Nut'tns	¼ cup	9	2	2	150
Super Soynuts, Unsalted	¼ cup	5	3	2	71
Super Soynuts, Craisinberry Crunch	¼ cup	9	7	2	53
The Fertile Hand Chocolate Pepitas (Chocolate Covered Pumpkin Seeds)	1 oz (28 g)	8	4	4	180
The Fertile Hand Extra Spicy Pepitas (Hot Garlic Roasted Pumpkin Seeds)	1 oz (28 g)	8	2	6	160
The Fertile Hand Nearly Naked (Lightly Salted Pumpkin Seeds)	1 oz (28 g)	6	2	4	180
The Fertile Hand Spicy Pepitas (Garlic Roasted Pumpkin Seeds)	1 oz (28 g)	6	2	4	180
The Fertile Hand Sweet Pepitas (Cinnamon Toasted Pumpkin Seeds)	1 oz (28 g)	12	5	7	150
NUT BUTTERS, GENERIC					
Almond butter	2 tbsp	6	4	2	202
Cashew butter	2 tbsp	8	8	2	186
Peanut butter, chunk style	2 tbsp	6	4	2	186
NUT BUTTERS, BY BRAND					
Atkins Beanit Butter	2 tbsp	5	1	5	170

FOOD	SERVING	TOTAL CARBS (G)	NET CARBS (G)	FIBER (G)	CALORIES
Atkins Macadamia Nut Butter	2 tbsp	5	2	na	230
Dixie Diners' Club Carb Not Beanit Butter	2 tbsp	5	0	5	170
Carb Options Creamy Peanut Butter	2 tbsp	5	3	2	190
Carb Options Super Chunky Peanut Butter	2 tbsp	5	3	2	190
ORGAN MEATS					
Brain, beef, simmered	4 oz	0	0	0	181
Brain, beef, pan fried	4 oz	0	0	0	222
Brain, pork, braised	4 oz	0	0	0	156
Giblets, fried	1 cup, chopped or diced	6	6	0	402
Sweetbread, braised	4 oz	0	0	0	362
Tripe, raw	4 oz	0	0	0	111
Tongue, beef, simmered	4 oz	t	t	0	321
Tongue, pork, simmered	4 oz	0	0	0	307
PANCAKES AND WAFFLES					
PANCAKES					
Blueberry pancakes, prepared from recipe	1 pancake (4" dia)	11	11	na	84
Blueberry pancakes, prepared from recipe	1 pancake (6" dia)	22	22	na	171
Buttermilk mini pancakes, frozen, ready to microwave	1 serving	22	22	na	116

PANCAKES AND WAFFLES

FOOD	SERVING	TOTAL CARBS (G)	NET CARBS (G)	FIBER (G)	CALORIES
Buttermilk pancakes, prepared from recipe	1 pancake (4" dia)	11	11	na	86
Buttermilk pancakes, prepared from recipe	1 pancake (6" dia)	22	22	na	175
Plain pancakes, dry mix, prepared	1 pancake (4" dia)	14	13.5	.5	74
Plain pancakes, dry mix, prepared	1 pancake (6" dia)	28	27	1	149
Plain pancakes, frozen, ready-to-heat	1 mini pancake	4	4	t	23
Plain pancakes, frozen, ready-to-heat	1 pancake (4" dia)	18	17	1	94
Plain pancakes, frozen, ready-to-heat	1 pancake (6" dia)	32	31	1	167
Plain pancakes, prepared from recipe	1 pancake (4" dia)	11	11	na	86
Plain pancakes, prepared from recipe	1 pancake (6" dia)	22	22	na	175
Whole-wheat pancakes, dry mix, prepared	1 pancake (4" dia)	13	12	1	92
Whole-wheat pancakes, dry mix, prepared	1 pancake (6" dia)	38	34	4	268
WAFFLES					
Banana bread waffles	1 serving	32	30	2	212
Buttermilk waffles, frozen, ready-to-heat	1 waffle (4" square)	15	14	1	98
Buttermilk waffles, frozen, ready-to-heat, toasted	1 waffle (4" dia)	13	12	1	87
Frozen waffles	1 serving	30	30	na	197

PANCAKES AND WAFFLES

FOOD	SERVING	TOTAL CARBS (G)	NET CARBS (G)	FIBER (G)	CALORIES
Oat waffles	1 waffle (4" dia)	13	12	1	69
Plain waffles	1 waffle (7" dia)	25	25	na	218
PANCAKE AND WAFFLE MIXES, BY BRAND, LOW CARB					
Atkins Quick Quisine Pancake & Waffle Mix	4 pancakes	6	3	3	80
Atkins Quick Quisine Deluxe Buttermilk Pancake & Waffle Mix	4 pancakes	13	8	5	100
CarboRite Low Carb Pancake Mix	3 pancakes (35 g)	10	4.8	t	100
Carbolite Pancake Mix	3 pancakes (35 g)	10	4.8	1	100
CarbSense Pancake & Waffle Mix	2 pancakes (38 g)	10	4	7	140
CarbSense Pancake & Waffle Mix, Buckwheat	2 pancakes (38 g)	10	3	7	140
CarbSense Pancake & Waffle Mix, Buttermilk	2 pancakes (38 g)	10	3	7	140
Flax-O-Meal Pancake & Waffle Mix, Apple Spice	2 pancakes	9	6	3	130
Flax-O-Meal Pancake & Waffle Mix, Banana Nut	2 pancakes	9	6	3	130
Ketogenics Low Carb Pancake Mix	2 pancakes (47 g)	15	5	6	185

284 PASTA AND NOODLES

FOOD	SERVING	TOTAL CARBS (G)	NET CARBS (G)	FIBER (G)	CALORIES
Keto Muffin & Pancake Mix, Banana	3 pancakes or 2 muffins	5	4	2	110
Keto Muffin & Pancake Mix, Blueberry	3 pancakes or 2 muffins	5	4	2	110
Keto Muffin & Pancake Mix, Golden Original	3 pancakes or 2 muffins	5	4	2	110
Labrada CarbWatchers Pancake & Waffle Mix	1 pancake (18 g)	12	4	6	80
Low Carb Success Flax-O-Meal Pancake & Waffle Mix, Butter Pecan	2 pancakes	9	4	3	140
MiniCarb Pancake Mix, Apple Cinnamon	2 pancakes (40 g)	7	3	6	150

PASTA AND NOODLES

PASTA AND NOODLES, GENERIC

FOOD	SERVING	TOTAL CARBS (G)	NET CARBS (G)	FIBER (G)	CALORIES
Alfredo egg noodles in creamy sauce, dry mix	1 serving	39	39	0	259
Chinese noodles, chow mein, cooked	½ cup	13	12	1	119
Corn pasta, cooked	½ cup	20	17	3	88
Egg noodles, enriched, cooked	½ cup	20	19	1	106
Egg noodles, spinach, enriched, cooked	½ cup	19	17	2	106
Fresh-refrigerated, plain	½ cup	28	28	na	149
Homemade, made w/o egg	½ cup	29	29	na	141

PASTA AND NOODLES

FOOD	SERVING	TOTAL CARBS (G)	NET CARBS (G)	FIBER (G)	CALORIES
Japanese noodles, soba, cooked	½ cup	12	12	na	56
Japanese noodles, somen, cooked	½ cup	24	24	na	115
Macaroni, elbow	½ cup	20	19	1	99
Macaroni, elbow, whole wheat, cooked	½ cup	19	17	2	87
Macaroni, spiral	½ cup	19	18	1	94
Macaroni, shells	½ cup	16	15	1	81
Pasta, w/sliced franks in tomato sauce, canned	1 serving	30	28	2	262
Spaghetti, w/salt	½ cup	20	19	1	99
Spinach pasta, refrigerated, cooked	½ cup	29	29	na	148
Spinach spaghetti, cooked	½ cup	18	18	na	9
Whole wheat spaghetti	½ cup	19	16	3	87
PASTA AND NOODLES, BY BRAND					
Aramana Cheddar Cheeseburger Pasta	1 cup	10	6	4	260
Aramana Creamy Chicken Alfredo Pasta	1 cup	11	6	5	260
Aramana Mild Mexican Chicken Pasta	1 cup	11	6	5	260
Atkins Quick Quisine Pasta Sides, Elbows & Cheese	1 cup	17	8	9	250
Atkins Quick Quisine Pasta Sides, Fettuccine Alfredo	1 cup	16	7	9	210

PASTA AND NOODLES

FOOD	SERVING	TOTAL CARBS (G)	NET CARBS (G)	FIBER (G)	CALORIES
Atkins Quick Quisine Pasta Sides, Pesto Cream	1 cup	17	7	10	240
Atkins Quick Quisine Penne	2 oz	13	5	8	210
Atkins Quick Quisine Rotini	2 oz	13	5	8	210
Atkins Quick Quisine Spaghetti	2 oz	13	5	8	210
Bella Vita Macaroni & Cheese	1 cup	17	11	6	291
Bella Vita Macaroni & White Cheddar	1 cup	17	11	6	291
Bella Vita Low Carb Pasta, Cavatappi	¾ cup	18	10	8	160
Bella Vita Low Carb Pasta, Elbows	¾ cup	18	10	8	160
Bella Vita Low Carb Pasta, Penne Rigate	¾ cup	18	10	8	160
Bella Vita Low Carb Pasta, Rigatoni	¾ cup	18	10	8	160
Bella Vita Low Carb Pasta, Rotini	¾ cup	18	10	8	160
Bella Vita Low Carb Pasta, Shells	¾ cup	18	10	8	160
Bella Vita Penne w/Creamy Alfredo Sauce	1 cup	17	11	6	296
Bella Vita Penne w/Roasted Garlic & Parmesan Spinach Sauce	1 cup	17	11	6	291

PASTA AND NOODLES

FOOD	SERVING	TOTAL CARBS (G)	NET CARBS (G)	FIBER (G)	CALORIES
Bella Vita Rotini w/Creamy Alfredo & Broccoli Sauce	1 cup	17	11	6	296
Bella Vita Rotini w/Roasted Garlic & Parmesan Sauce	1 cup	17	11	6	291
Darielle Pasta Elbows	¾ cup	18	10	8	160
Darielle Pasta Fusilli	¾ cup	18	10	8	160
Darielle Pasta Mezze Penne	¾ cup	18	10	8	160
Darielle Pasta Penne	¾ cup	18	10	8	160
Dixie Diners' Club Skinni Spaghetti	2 oz	14	3	11	143
Keto Pasta Elbows	1.3 oz (dry)	7	5	2	130
Keto Pasta Fettuccine	1.3 oz (dry)	7	5	2	130
Keto Pasta Macaroni & Cheese	1.7 oz (dry)	7	5	2	130
Keto Pasta Shells	¾ cup (dry)	7	5	2	130
Keto Pasta Spaghetti	¾ cup (dry)	7	5	2	130
Ketogenics Mac N Cheese	1.5 oz	11	6.5	4.5	325
Pastalia Fettuccine	2 oz	10	7	3	176
Pastalia Fettuccine Tomato Basil	2 oz	10	7	3	176
Pastalia Low Carb Pasta	2 oz	10	7	3	176
Pastalia Tomato Basil Low Carb Pasta	2 oz	10	7	3	176
Whey Cool Macaroni & Cheese Dinner	1 cup	12	11	1	260

PASTRIES AND DONUTS

FOOD	SERVING	TOTAL CARBS (G)	NET CARBS (G)	FIBER (G)	CALORIES
Whey Cool Xtreme Pasta	2 oz	8	7	1	210

PASTRIES AND DONUTS

PASTRIES AND DONUTS, BY BRAND

FOOD	SERVING	TOTAL CARBS (G)	NET CARBS (G)	FIBER (G)	CALORIES
Atkins Chocolate Glazed Donut Mix	1 donut	10	2	8	60
Atkins Rugelach, Apricot	5 pieces (1 oz)	5	3	2	180
Atkins Rugelach, Chocolate	5 pieces (1 oz)	7	5	2	170
Atkins Rugelach, Raspberry	5 pieces (1 oz)	5	3	2	180
Atkins French Crepe Mix	1 crepe, dry (5.5 g)	2	t	2	12
CarboRite Blueberry Toaster Tart	1 tart	26	6	8	130
CarboRite Cinnamon Toaster Tart	1 tart	26	6	8	140
CarboRite Strawberry Toaster Tart	1 tart	26	6	8	130

DONUTS, GENERIC

FOOD	SERVING	TOTAL CARBS (G)	NET CARBS (G)	FIBER (G)	CALORIES
Cake type, wheat, sugared or glazed	1 donut, medium (3" dia)	19	18	1	162
Cake type, wheat, sugared or glazed	1 donut (2" dia)	12	11	1	101
Cake type, plain, sugared or glazed	1 donut, medium (3" dia)	23	22	1	192
Cake type, plain, chocolate-coated or frosted	1 donut, large (3½" dia)	27	26	1	270

PASTRIES AND DONUTS 289

FOOD	SERVING	TOTAL CARBS (G)	NET CARBS (G)	FIBER (G)	CALORIES
Cake type, plain, chocolate-coated or frosted	1 donut, medium (3" dia)	21	20	1	204
Cake type, plain, chocolate-coated or frosted	1 donut (2" dia)	13	12	1	133
Cake type, plain, unsugared, old fashioned	1 donut stick	26	25	1	219
Cake type, plain, unsugared, old fashioned	1 donut, large (4" dia)	35	34	1	299
Cake type, plain, unsugared, old fashioned	1 donut, mini (1½" dia or donut hole)	7	7	t	59
Cake type, plain, unsugared, old fashioned	1 donut, medium (3¼" dia)	23	22	1	198
Cake type, plain, unsugared, old fashioned	1 donut, long type (twist, 4½" long)	26	25	1	219
Cake type, chocolate, sugared or glazed	1 donut, medium (3" dia)	24	23	1	175
Cake type, chocolate, sugared or glazed	1 donut (3¾" dia)	34	33	1	250
Donut stick, cake type, plain	1 donut stick	26	25	1	219
Donut stick, yeast leavened, glazed, enriched	1 donut stick	25	24	1	226

PASTRIES AND DONUTS

FOOD	SERVING	TOTAL CARBS (G)	NET CARBS (G)	FIBER (G)	CALORIES
Donut twist, yeast leavened, glazed, enriched	1 donut twist (4½")	26	25	1	219
Donut hole, yeast leavened, glazed, enriched	1 donut hole	6	6	t	52
French crullers, glazed	1 cruller (3" dia)	24	23	1	169
Yeast leavened, w/crème filling	1 donut oval (3½" x 2½")	26	25	1	307
Yeast leavened, w/jelly filling	1 donut oval (3½" x 2½")	33	32	1	289
PASTRIES, GENERIC					
Apple turnovers, frozen, ready to bake	1 serving	31	29	2	284
Cream puffs, prepared from recipe	1 cream puff	30	30	t	335
Coffee cake, cheese	1 piece (⅙ of 16 oz cake)	34	33	1	258
Coffee cake, cinnamon w/crumb topping, commercially prepared	1 piece (⅑ of 20 oz cake)	29	28	1	263
Coffee cake, crème-filled w/chocolate frosting	1 piece (⅙ of 19 oz cake)	48	46	2	298
Coffee cake, fruit	1 piece (⅛ cake)	26	25	1	156
Croissant, apple	1 croissant, medium	21	20	1	145
Croissant, butter	1 croissant, large	31	29	2	272
Croissant, butter	1 croissant, medium	26	25	1	231
Croissant, butter	1 croissant, small	19	18	1	171
Croissant, butter	1 croissant, mini	13	12	1	114

PASTRIES AND DONUTS

FOOD	SERVING	TOTAL CARBS (G)	NET CARBS (G)	FIBER (G)	CALORIES
Croissant, cheese	1 croissant, large	31	29	2	277
Croissant, cheese	1 croissant, medium	27	25	2	236
Croissant, cheese	1 croissant, small	20	19	1	174
Croissant, cheese	1 croissant, mini	13	12	1	114
Danish pastry, cheese	1 pastry	26	25	1	266
Danish pastry, cinnamon	1 pastry, large (7" dia)	63	61	2	572
Danish pastry, cinnamon	1 pastry (4¼" dia)	29	28	1	262
Danish pastry, cinnamon	1 pastry, small or frozen (3" dia)	16	16	t	141
Danish pastry, cinnamon	1 piece (⅛ of 15 oz ring)	24	23	1	214
Danish pastry, fruit	1 pastry, large (7" dia)	68	65	3	527
Danish pastry, fruit	1 pastry (4¼" dia)	34	33	1	262
Danish pastry, fruit	1 pastry, small or frozen (3" dia)	17	16	1	130
Danish pastry, fruit	1 piece (⅛ of 15 oz ring)	25	24	1	197
Danish pastry, nut	1 pastry (4¼" dia)	30	29	1	280
Danish pastry, nut	1 piece (⅛ of 15 oz ring)	24	23	1	228
Éclairs, custard-filled w/chocolate glaze, prepared from recipe	1 small éclair, (3½" x 2")	27	26	1	293
Éclairs, custard-filled w/chocolate glaze, prepared from recipe	1 medium éclair, (5" x 2" x 1¾")	24	23	1	262

PASTRIES AND DONUTS

FOOD	SERVING	TOTAL CARBS (G)	NET CARBS (G)	FIBER (G)	CALORIES
Sweet rolls, cinnamon, refrigerated dough w/frosting, baked	1 roll	17	17	na	109
Sweet rolls, cinnamon, refrigerated dough w/frosting	1 roll	15	15	na	100
Sweet rolls, cinnamon, commercially prepared w/raisins	1 roll (2¾" square)	31	30	1	223
Sweet rolls, cinnamon, commercially prepared w/raisins	1 roll, large	42	40	2	309
Sweet rolls, cheese	1 roll	29	28	1	238
Toaster pastry, apple cinnamon	1 pastry	37	36	1	205
Toaster pastry, apple cinnamon Danish swirl	1 pastry	37	36	1	256
Toaster pastry, blueberry blueberry	1 pastry	36	35	1	212
Toaster pastry, blueberry, frosted	1 pastry	37	36	1	203
Toaster pastry, frosted chocolate fudge, low fat	1 pastry	40	39	1	190
Toaster pastry, brown sugar & cinnamon	1 pastry	34	33	1	206
Toaster pastry, brown sugar & cinnamon, frosted	1 pastry	34	33	1	211

FOOD	SERVING	TOTAL CARBS (G)	NET CARBS (G)	FIBER (G)	CALORIES
Toaster pastry, cheese Danish	1 pastry	37	37	t	252
Toaster pastry, cherry	1 pastry	37	36	1	204
Toaster pastry, cherry, frosted	1 pastry	37	37	t	204
Toaster pastry, chocolate fudge, frosted	1 pastry	37	37	1	201
Toaster pastry, chocolate vanilla crème, frosted	1 pastry	37	36	1	203
Toaster pastry, fruit	1 pastry	37	36	1	204
Toaster pastry, grape, frosted	1 pastry	38	37	1	203
Toaster pastry, milk chocolate	1 pastry	36	35	1	205
Toaster pastry, raspberry, frosted	1 pastry	37	36	1	205
Toaster pastry, strawberry Danish	1 pastry	37	36	1	254
Toaster pastry, strawberry, frosted	1 pastry	37	36	1	203
Toaster pastry, strudel	1 pastry	24	23	1	214
Toaster pastry, wild berry, frosted	1 pastry	39	38	1	210

PICKLES AND OLIVES

FOOD	SERVING	TOTAL CARBS (G)	NET CARBS (G)	FIBER (G)	CALORIES
Dill pickle	1 spear	1	1	t	5
Dill pickle, chopped	½ cup	3	2	1	13
Dill pickle, large	1 pickle (4" long)	6	4	2	24
Dill pickle, medium	1 pickle (3¾" long)	3	2	1	12
Dill pickle, small	1 pickle	2	2	t	7

294 PIES AND PIE FILLINGS

FOOD	SERVING	TOTAL CARBS (G)	NET CARBS (G)	FIBER (G)	CALORIES
Sour pickle	1 spear	1	1	t	3
Sour pickle, chopped	½ cup	2	1	1	36
Sour pickle, large	1 pickle (4" long)	3	1	2	15
Sour pickle, medium	1 pickle (3¾" long)	1	0	1	7
Sour pickle, small	1 pickle	1	1	t	4
Sweet pickle (gherkin)	1 spear	6	6	t	23
Sweet pickle, chopped	½ cup	25	24	1	94
Sweet pickle (gherkin), large	1 pickle (4" long)	11	11	t	41
Sweet pickle (gherkin), medium	1 pickle (2¾" long)	8	8	t	29
Sweet pickle (gherkin), midget	1 pickle (2⅛" long)	2	2	t	7
Sweet pickle (gherkin), small	1 pickle (2½" long)	5	5	t	18
Olive, green	5 olives	t	t	na	23
Olives, ripe, canned, colossal	1 olive	1	1	t	12
Olives, ripe, canned, jumbo	1 olive	t	t	t	7
Olives, ripe, canned, large	1 olive	t	t	t	5
Olives, ripe, canned, small	1 olive	t	t	t	4

PIES AND PIE FILLINGS

FOOD	SERVING	TOTAL CARBS (G)	NET CARBS (G)	FIBER (G)	CALORIES
Apple pie, frozen, ready to bake	1 serving	41	40	1	292
Apple, commercially prepared, enriched flour	1 piece (⅙ of 9" dia)	43	41	2	296

PIES AND PIE FILLINGS

FOOD	SERVING	TOTAL CARBS (G)	NET CARBS (G)	FIBER (G)	CALORIES
Apple, commercially prepared, enriched flour	1 piece (⅙ of 8" dia)	40	38	2	277
Apple, prepared from recipe	1 piece (⅛ of 9" dia)	58	58	na	411
Banana cream, prepared from recipe	1 piece (⅛ of 9" dia)	47	46	1	387
Blueberry, commercially prepared	1 piece (⅙ of 8" dia)	41	40	1	271
Blueberry, prepared from recipe	1 piece (⅛ of 9" dia)	49	49	na	360
Boston cream pie, commercially prepared	1 piece (⅙ of 8" dia)	39	38	1	232
Cherry, commercially prepared	1 piece (⅛ of 9" dia)	50	49	1	325
Cherry, commercially prepared	1 piece (⅙ of 8" dia)	47	46	1	304
Cherry, prepared from recipe	1 piece (⅛ of 9" dia)	69	69	na	486
Chocolate crème, commercially prepared	1 piece (⅙ of 8" dia)	38	36	2	344
Chocolate mousse, prepared from mix, no-bake type	1 piece (⅛ of 9" dia)	28	28	na	247
Coconut cream, prepared from mix, no-bake type	1 piece (⅛ of 9" dia)	27	26	1	259
Coconut cream, commercially prepared	1 piece (⅛ of 7" dia)	18	17	1	143

PIES AND PIE FILLINGS

FOOD	SERVING	TOTAL CARBS (G)	NET CARBS (G)	FIBER (G)	CALORIES
Coconut custard, commercially prepared	1 piece (⅙ of 8" dia)	31	29	2	270
Egg custard, commercially prepared	1 piece (⅙ of 8" dia)	22	20	2	221
Fried pie, cherry	1 pie (5" x 3¾")	55	52	3	404
Fried pie, fruit	1 pie (5" x 3¾")	55	52	3	404
Fried pie, lemon	1 pie (5" x 3¾")	55	52	3	404
Lemon meringue, commercially prepared	1 piece (⅙ of 8" dia)	53	52	1	303
Lemon meringue, prepared from recipe	1 piece (⅛ of 9" dia)	50	50	na	362
Mince, prepared from recipe	1 piece (⅛ of 9" dia)	79	75	4	477
Peach	1 piece (⅙ of 8" dia)	38	36	1	261
Pecan, commercially prepared	1 piece (⅙ of 8" dia)	65	61	4	452
Pecan, prepared from recipe	1 piece (⅛ of 9" dia)	64	64	na	503
Pumpkin, commercially prepared	1 piece (⅙ of 8" dia)	30	27	3	229
Pumpkin, prepared from recipe	1 piece (⅛ of 9" dia)	41	41	na	316
Vanilla cream, prepared from recipe	1 piece (⅛ of 9" dia)	41	40	1	350
PIE FILLINGS					
Steel's Apple Pie Filling	⅓ cup (85 g)	6.5	.2	1.3	25

FOOD	SERVING	TOTAL CARBS (G)	NET CARBS (G)	FIBER (G)	CALORIES
Steel's Blueberry Pie Filling	⅓ cup (85 g)	7.4	.5	1.5	34
Steel's Cherry Pie Filling	⅓ cup (85 g)	6	0	1	25
Steel's Peach Pie Filling	⅓ cup (85 g)	4.5	0	.5	17

PIZZAS

PIZZAS,* GENERIC

FOOD	SERVING	TOTAL CARBS (G)	NET CARBS (G)	FIBER (G)	CALORIES
Cheese, whole pizza	1 pizza (12" dia)	164	164	na	1,122
Cheese, slice	1 slice	21	21	0	140
Cheese, meat, & vegetables, whole pizza	1 pizza (12" dia)	170	170	na	1,470
Cheese, meat, & vegetables, slice	1 slice	21	21	na	184
Cheese, sausage, pepperoni & onions, frozen, whole pizza	1 package	166	166	na	1,746
Cheese, sausage, pepperoni & onions, frozen	1 serving	32	32	na	337
Crispy crust pepperoni, frozen, whole pizza	1 package	69	69	na	728
Crispy crust pepperoni, frozen	1 serving	35	35	na	364
Deep-dish sausage pizza, frozen, whole pizza	1 package	164	164	na	1,576
Deep-dish sausage pizza, frozen	1 serving	41	41	na	391
French bread pizza w/ sausage & pepperoni, frozen, whole pizza	1 package	87	82	5	896

* Includes values for whole pizza and individual serving sizes.

PIZZAS

FOOD	SERVING	TOTAL CARBS (G)	NET CARBS (G)	FIBER (G)	CALORIES
French bread pizza w/ sausage & pepperoni, frozen	1 serving	44	41.5	2.5	448
French bread pizza w/ sausage, pepperoni & mushrooms, frozen, whole pizza	1 package	89	82	7	858
French bread pizza w/ sausage, pepperoni & mushrooms, frozen	1 serving	44	40.5	3.5	429
Mexican-style pizza, frozen, whole pizza	1 package	130	130	na	1,326
Mexican-style pizza, frozen	1 serving	43	43	na	437
Pepperoni, frozen, whole pizza	1 package	118	118	na	1,288
Pepperoni, frozen	1 serving	36	34	2	400
Pepperoni, whole pizza	1 pizza (12" dia)	159	159	na	1,446
Pepperoni, slice	1 slice	20	20	na	181
Pepperoni, stuffed sandwich, frozen	1 serving	39	39	na	367
Pizza snacks, hamburger, frozen	1 serving	26	26	na	231
Pizza snacks, pepperoni, frozen	1 serving	39	37	2	385
Pizza snacks, sausage, frozen	1 serving	40	37	3	351
Sausage, green & red peppers, mushroom, frozen, whole pizza	1 package	133	133	na	1,538

FOOD	SERVING	TOTAL CARBS (G)	NET CARBS (G)	FIBER (G)	CALORIES
Sausage, green & red peppers, mushroom, frozen	1 serving	33	33	na	386
Sausage & mushroom frozen, whole pizza	1 package	152	152	na	1,496
Sausage & mushroom frozen	1 serving	31	31	na	306
Sausage, mushrooms & pepperoni, frozen, whole pizza	1 package	160	160	na	1,736
Sausage, mushrooms & pepperoni, frozen	1 serving	32	32	na	344
Sausage & pepperoni, frozen, whole pizza	1 package	120	120	na	1,389
Sausage & pepperoni, frozen	1 serving	30	30	na	348
PIZZA MIXES, BY BRAND					
Atkins Quick Quisine Smokehouse Pizza	1 serving	22	11	11	420
Atkins Quick Quisine Supreme Pizza	1 serving	22	11	11	360
CarbSense Pizza Crust Mix, Garlic & Herb	1 slice	7	3	4	100
LowCarbolicious Pizza Kit, Crust Only	12" pizza	25	24	1	389
LowCarbolicious Pizza Kit, Sauce Only	12" pizza	7	6	1	65
Low Carb Success Flax-O-Meal Pizza Crust	1 slice	7	3	4	130

FOOD	SERVING	TOTAL CARBS (G)	NET CARBS (G)	FIBER (G)	CALORIES
Keto Pizza Dough	1 slice (22 g)	4.5	2	2.5	80
MiniCarb Pizza Crust Mix, Parmesan Herb	1 slice (28 g)	5	2	3	130

PORK, HAM, AND BACON

PORK, LEAN CUTS

FOOD	SERVING	TOTAL CARBS (G)	NET CARBS (G)	FIBER (G)	CALORIES
Center loin chop, w/bone, lean only, braised	4 oz edible portion	0	0	0	229
Center loin chop, w/bone, lean only, broiled	4 oz edible portion	0	0	0	229
Sirloin chop, w/bone, lean only, braised	4 oz edible portion	0	0	0	223
Sirloin chop, boneless, lean only, broiled	4 oz	0	0	0	219
Sirloin roast, boneless, lean only, roasted	4 oz	0	0	0	224
Tenderloin, lean only, broiled	4 oz	0	0	0	212
Tenderloin, lean only, roasted	4 oz	0	0	0	186
Tenderloin, lean & fat, broiled	4 oz	0	0	0	228
Top loin chop, boneless, lean only, braised	4 oz	0	0	0	229
Top loin chop, boneless, lean only, braised	4 oz	0	0	0	230

VARIETY MEATS, LEAN

FOOD	SERVING	TOTAL CARBS (G)	NET CARBS (G)	FIBER (G)	CALORIES
Pork heart, braised	1 heart	.5	.5	0	191
Pork kidneys, braised	4 oz	0	0	0	171

FOOD	SERVING	TOTAL CARBS (G)	NET CARBS (G)	FIBER (G)	CALORIES
Pork liver, braised	4 oz	4	4	0	187
Pork spleen, braised	4 oz	0	0	0	169

PORK PRODUCTS

PORK

FOOD	SERVING	TOTAL CARBS (G)	NET CARBS (G)	FIBER (G)	CALORIES
Boston blade, roasted	4 oz	0	0	0	304
Ham, cured, whole, roasted	4 oz	0	0	0	275
Ham, patties, grilled	1 patty, cooked	1	1	0	205
Cutlet, cooked	4 oz	0	0	0	284
Ground, cooked	4 oz	0	0	0	336
Loin blade (chops), bone in, lean & fat only, braised	4 oz	0	0	0	366
Loin blade (chops), bone in, lean & fat only, broiled	4 oz	0	0	0	363
Loin blade (chops), bone in, lean & fat only, pan fried	4 oz	0	0	0	388
Loin blade (chops), bone in, lean & fat only, roasted	4 oz	0	0	0	366
Loin, country-style ribs, lean & fat only, braised	4 oz	0	0	0	335
Loin, country-style ribs, lean & fat only, roasted	4 oz	0	0	0	372
Shoulder, arm picnic, lean & fat only, braised	4 oz	0	0	0	373

POULTRY

FOOD	SERVING	TOTAL CARBS (G)	NET CARBS (G)	FIBER (G)	CALORIES
Shoulder, arm picnic, lean & fat only, roasted	4 oz	0	0	0	359
Shoulder, blade roll, lean & fat only, roasted	4 oz	t	t	0	325
Spareribs, cooked	4 oz	0	0	0	448
BACON					
Bacon, Canadian style, grilled	2 slices	1	1	0	87
Bacon, fried, drained	3 slices	t	t	0	108
Bacon, meatless	2 strips	1	1	t	31
Bacon, turkey	1 serving	t	t	0	35
POULTRY					
CHICKEN					
Breast, meat only, roasted broiler or fryer	4 oz	0	0	0	186
Chicken w/skin, roasted	4 oz	0	0	0	272
Chicken, dark meat, w/skin, roasted	4 oz	0	0	0	288
Chicken, dark meat, w/skin, fried in batter	4 oz	11	11	na	334
Chicken, dark meat, w/skin, fried in flour	4 oz	5	5	na	319
Chicken breast, broiler or fryer, meat & skin, fried in batter	½ breast	13	13	t	364

FOOD	SERVING	TOTAL CARBS (G)	NET CARBS (G)	FIBER (G)	CALORIES
Chicken breast, broiler or fryer, meat & skin, fried in flour	½ breast	2	2	t	218
Chicken drumstick, broiler or fryer, meat & skin, fried in batter	1 drumstick, bone removed	6	6	t	193
Chicken drumstick, broiler or fryer, meat & skin, fried in flour	1 drumstick, bone removed	1	1	0	120
Chicken wing, broiler or fryer, meat & skin, fried in batter	1 wing, bone removed	5	5	t	159
Chicken wing, broiler or fryer, meat & skin, fried in flour	1 wing, bone removed	1	1	0	103
Dark meat, roasted, broiler or fryer	4 oz	0	0	0	232
Dark meat, roasted, roaster	4 oz	0	0	0	201
Drumstick, meat only, roasted, broiler or fryer	4 oz	0	0	0	194
Drumstick, meat only, roasted, broiler or fryer	1 drumstick	0	0	0	76
Leg, meat only, roasted, broiler or fryer	1 leg	0	0	0	181
Light meat, roasted, broiler or fryer	4 oz	0	0	0	195

POULTRY

FOOD	SERVING	TOTAL CARBS (G)	NET CARBS (G)	FIBER (G)	CALORIES
Light meat, roasted, roaster	4 oz	0	0	0	173
Light meat, stewed, stewer	4 oz	0	0	0	241
Wing, meat only, roasted, broiler or fryer	1 wing	0	0	0	43
DUCK AND GOOSE					
Duck, meat & skin, roasted	4 oz	0	0	0	377
Duck, wild, breast, w/o skin, cooked	4 oz	0	0	0	140
Goose, domesticated, meat & skin, roasted	4 oz	0	0	0	342
Goose, w/o skin, roasted	4 oz	0	0	0	268
VARIETY AND SPECIALTY POULTRY					
Cornish game hen, meat only, roasted	½ hen	0	0	0	147
Cornish game hens, meat & skin, roasted	½ bird	0	0	0	335
Liver, chicken, cooked	4 oz	0	0	0	176
Ostrich, cooked	4 oz	0	0	0	160
Pâté de foie gras, (goose liver pâté), canned, smoked	1 tbsp	1	1	0	60
Pheasant, w/o skin, cooked	4 oz	0	0	0	152

TURKEY

FOOD	SERVING	TOTAL CARBS (G)	NET CARBS (G)	FIBER (G)	CALORIES
Back meat, w/o skin, roasted	4 oz	0	0	0	192
Boneless, roast, light & dark meat	4 oz	3	3	0	175
Breast meat, w/o skin, roasted	4 oz	0	0	0	153
Canned, meat only, w/broth	4 oz	0	0	0	184
Dark meat, roasted	4 oz	0	0	0	183
Ground turkey	1 patty, 4 oz	0	0	0	193
Leg meat, w/o skin, roasted	4 oz	0	0	0	180
Light meat, all classes, roasted	4 oz	0	0	0	177
Meat, all classes, roasted	4 oz	0	0	0	192
Neck meat, w/o skin, cooked	4 oz	0	0	0	203
Turkey breast, meat & skin, roasted	4 oz	0	0	0	141
Turkey, canned	1 can (5 oz)	0	0	0	204
Turkey dark meat, meat & skin, roasted	1 cup	0	0	0	309
Turkey w/gravy, frozen	1 pkg	7	7	0	95
Turkey ham	4 oz	4	4	0	134
Turkey leg, meat & skin, roasted	½ leg	0	0	0	568
Turkey light meat, meat & skin, roasted	1 cup	0	0	0	276

PUDDINGS

FOOD	SERVING	TOTAL CARBS (G)	NET CARBS (G)	FIBER (G)	CALORIES
Turkey patties, battered, fried	1 patty	10	10	t	181
Turkey sticks, battered & fried	2 sticks	22	22	na	357
Turkey wing, meat & skin, roasted	1 wing, bone removed	0	0	0	426
Wing, w/o skin & bone	1 wing	0	0	0	98
Young hen, dark meat, w/o skin, roasted	4 oz	0	0	0	217
Young hen, light meat, w/o skin, roasted	4 oz	0	0	0	182
Young hen, meat only, roasted	4 oz	0	0	0	198
Young tom, dark meat, w/o skin, roasted	4 oz	0	0	0	209
Young tom, light meat, w/o skin, roasted	4 oz	0	0	0	174
Young tom, meat, w/o skin, roasted	4 oz	0	0	0	190

PUDDINGS

PUDDINGS, GENERIC

FOOD	SERVING	TOTAL CARBS (G)	NET CARBS (G)	FIBER (G)	CALORIES
Banana, dry mix, instant	1 portion, makes ½ cup	23	23	0	92
Banana, dry mix, instant, w/added oil	1 portion, makes ½ cup	22	22	0	97
Banana, dry mix, regular	1 portion, makes ½ cup	20	20	t	83
Banana, dry mix, regular, w/added oil	1 portion, makes ½ cup	19	19	t	85
Banana, ready-to-eat	1 can (5 oz)	30	30	t	180

PUDDINGS

FOOD	SERVING	TOTAL CARBS (G)	NET CARBS (G)	FIBER (G)	CALORIES
Chocolate, dry mix, instant	1 portion, makes ½ cup	22	21	1	89
Chocolate, dry mix, regular	1 portion, makes ½ cup	22	21.5	.5	90
Chocolate, ready-to-eat	1 can (5 oz)	32	31	1	189
Chocolate, ready-to-eat	1 snack size (4 oz)	26	25	1	150
Coconut cream, dry mix, instant	1 portion, makes ½ cup	22	22	t	97
Coconut cream, dry mix, regular	1 portion, makes ½ cup	22	22	t	98
Lemon, dry mix, instant	1 portion, makes ½ cup	24	24	0	95
Lemon, dry mix, regular	1 portion, makes ½ cup	19	19	0	76
Lemon, ready-to-eat	1 can (5 oz)	36	36	t	178
Rice, dry mix	1 portion, makes ½ cup	25	25	t	102
Rice, ready-to-eat	1 can (5 oz)	31	31	t	231
Tapioca, dry milk	1 portion, makes ½ cup	22	22	0	85
Tapioca, ready-to-eat	1 can (5 oz)	28	28	t	169
Tapioca, ready-to-eat	1 snack size (4 oz)	22	22	t	134
Vanilla, dry mix, instant	1 portion, makes ½ cup	23	23	0	92
Vanilla, dry mix, regular	1 portion, makes ½ cup	21	21	t	81
Vanilla, ready-to-eat	1 snack size (4 oz)	25	25	t	147
PUDDINGS, BY BRAND					
Atkins Make-Your-Own Pudding Mix, Chocolate	½ cup (6.6 g)	4	1	3	26

SALAD DRESSINGS

FOOD	SERVING	TOTAL CARBS (G)	NET CARBS (G)	FIBER (G)	CALORIES
Atkins Make-Your-Own Pudding Mix, Vanilla	½ cup (6.6 g)	2	1	1	21
Dixie Diners' Club Chocolate Pudding Mix	½ cup	3	1	2	92
Dixie Diners' Club Vanilla Pudding Mix	½ cup	2	1	1	104
Expert Foods Wise CHOice Cook-It-Up Pudding Mix	½ tbsp dry mix for 1 serving	1.6	.1	1.5	145
Keto Pudding Mix, Banana	½ scoop dry mix for 1 serving	3	1	2	110
Keto Pudding Mix, Chocolate	½ scoop dry mix for 1 serving	4	1	3	110
Keto Pudding Mix, French Vanilla	½ scoop dry mix for 1 serving	3	1	2	110
SALAD DRESSINGS					
Bacon Ranch	2 tbsp	0	0	0	0
Creamy Bacon (Walden Farms)	2 tbsp	0	0	0	0
Creamy Bacon, in Packets (Walden Farms)	1 oz pkt	0	0	0	0
Bleu Cheese (Walden Farms)	2 tbsp	0	0	0	0
Blue cheese, regular	1 tbsp	2	2	0	60
Blue cheese, low fat	2 tbsp	4	4	0	60
Blue Cheese Dressing (Carb Options)	2 tbsp	0	0	0	150

SALAD DRESSINGS

FOOD	SERVING	TOTAL CARBS (G)	NET CARBS (G)	FIBER (G)	CALORIES
Caesar (Walden Farms)	2 tbsp	0	0	0	0
Caesar salad dressing, low calorie	2 tbsp	6	6	0	32
Coleslaw dressing, reduced fat	2 tbsp	14	14	0	112
Country French (Atkins)	1 oz	1	1	0	100
Country Italian (Walden Farms)	2 tbsp	0	0	0	0
Creamy Ranch (Atkins)	2 tbsp	1	1	0	110
French, regular	1 tbsp	3	3	0	69
French (Carb Options)	2 tbsp	1	1	t	100
French (Walden Farms)	2 tbsp	0	0	0	0
French, diet, low fat	2 tbsp	7	7	0	43
Honey Dijon (Walden Farms)	1 oz pkt	0	0	0	0
Honey Dijon Vinaigrette (Walden Farms)	2 tbsp	0	0	0	0
Honey Mustard, Sugar Free (Steel's)	1 tbsp	0	0	0	90
Italian, regular	1 tbsp	2	2	0	69
Italian, diet	2 tbsp	1	1	0	32
Italian, Fat Free (Kraft)	2 tbsp	4	4	t	20
Italian (Carb Options)	2 tbsp	0	0	0	70
Italian, Light Done Right (Kraft)	2 tbsp	2	2	t	53
Italian, Zesty (Kraft)	1 tbsp	1	1	t	54

SALAD DRESSINGS

FOOD	SERVING	TOTAL CARBS (G)	NET CARBS (G)	FIBER (G)	CALORIES
Italian (Walden Farms)	2 tbsp	0	0	0	0
Lemon Poppyseed (Atkins)	1 oz	1	1	0	100
Olive oil vinaigrette	2 tbsp	0	0	0	50
Oriental (Walden Farms)	2 tbsp	0	0	0	0
Ranch, Regular (Kraft)	1 tbsp	t	t	0	74
Ranch, Fat Free (Kraft)	2 tbsp	11	11	t	48
Ranch (Carb Options)	2 tbsp	0	0	0	150
Ranch, Light Done Right (Kraft)	2 tbsp	3	3	t	77
Ranch (Walden Farms)	2 tbsp	0	0	0	0
Ranch (Walden Farms)	1 oz pkt	0	0	0	0
Russian, regular	1 tbsp	2	0	3	74
Russian, low calorie	2 tbsp	9	9	t	45
Russian (Walden Farms)	2 tbsp	0	0	0	0
Sesame seed dressing	1 tbsp	1	1	t	66
Sweet As Honey Mustard Dressing (Atkins)	1 oz	1	1	0	110
Thousand Island, regular	1 tbsp	2	2	0	60
Thousand Island, low calorie, diet	2 tbsp	5	5	t	48
Thousand Island (Walden Farms)	2 tbsp	0	0	0	0
Thousand Island (Walden Farms)	1 oz pkt	0	0	0	0
Vinaigrette, balsamic	1 tbsp	2	2	0	50

SAUCES, GRAVIES, AND MARINADES

FOOD	SERVING	TOTAL CARBS (G)	NET CARBS (G)	FIBER (G)	CALORIES
Vinaigrette, Balsamic, Zero Calorie (Walden Farms)	2 tbsp	0	0	0	0
Vinaigrette, Balsamic, No Carbs (Walden Farms)	2 tbsp	0	0	0	40
Vinaigrette, Raspberry (Walden Farms)	2 tbsp	0	0	0	0
Vinaigrette, Red Wine (Walden Farms)	2 tbsp	0	0	0	0
Vinaigrette, red wine	1 tbsp	1	1	na	45
SAUCES, GRAVIES, AND MARINADES					
SAUCES, GENERIC					
Adobo fresco	1 tbsp	3	3	0	41
Barbecue sauce	2 tbsp	4	4	t	24
Barbecue sauce, hickory smoke	2 tbsp	9	9	t	39
Béarnaise, dehydrated, dry	1 pkt	15	15	0	91
Cheese sauce, ready-to-serve	¼ cup	4	4	t	110
Golden cheese sauce, ready-to-serve	¼ cup	2	1	1	139
Creole sauce, ready-to-serve	¼ cup	4	3	1	25
Fish sauce, ready-to-serve	2 tbsp	1	1	0	13
Hoisin sauce, ready-to-serve	2 tbsp	14	13	1	70

SAUCES, GRAVIES, AND MARINADES

FOOD	SERVING	TOTAL CARBS (G)	NET CARBS (G)	FIBER (G)	CALORIES
Hollandaise, w/ butterfat, dehydrated, prepared w/water	1 pkt	44	43	1	188
Jalapeño cheese sauce, ready-to-serve	¼ cup	8	8	0	81
Lemon sauce, ready-to-serve	2 tbsp	10	10	0	43
Mild nacho cheese sauce, ready-to-serve	¼ cup	3	2.5	.5	119
Nacho cheese sauce, ready-to-serve	¼ cup	4	4	t	128
Nacho cheese sauce, w/jalapeño peppers, mild, ready-to-serve	¼ cup	7	7	t	122
Plum sauce, ready-to-serve	2 tbsp	16	16	t	70
Sharp cheddar cheese sauce, ready-to-serve	¼ cup	2	1	1	133
Stir fry sauce, ready-to-serve	1 tbsp	2	2	0	16
Sweet & sour sauce, dry	1 pkt	55	55	1	222
Sweet & sour glaze, ready-to-serve	2 tbsp	12	12	0	51
Sweet & sour sauce, ready-to-serve	2 tbsp	8	8	t	40
Tartar sauce	1 tbsp	2	2	0	74
White sauce, homemade, thin	¼ cup	5	5	t	66
White sauce, homemade, medium	¼ cup	6	6	t	92

SAUCES, GRAVIES, AND MARINADES 313

FOOD	SERVING	TOTAL CARBS (G)	NET CARBS (G)	FIBER (G)	CALORIES
White sauce, homemade, thick	¼ cup	7	7	t	116
SAUCES, BY BRAND, LOW CARB					
Atkins Barbecue Sauce	1 tbsp	0	0	na	15
Atkins Quick Quisine Steak Sauce & Marinade	1 tbsp	1	1	0	5
Atkins Quick Quisine Teriyaki Sauce & Marinade	1 tbsp	1	1	0	10
Steel's Rocky Mountain Barbecue Sauce, Original	2 tbsp	10	4.5	0	35
Carb Options Alfredo Sauce	¼ cup	2	2	0	110
Carb Options Asian Teriyaki Marinade	1 tbsp	1	1	0	5
Carb Options Double Cheddar Sauce	¼ cup	2	2	0	90
Carb Options Garden Style Sauce	½ cup	7	5	2	80
Carb Options Hickory Barbecue Sauce	2 tbsp	3	3	0	10
Carb Options Hearty Italian Style Pasta Sauce w/Sausage	½ cup	7	5	2	160
Carb Options Italian Garlic Marinade	1 tbsp	0	0	0	0
Carb Options Original Barbecue Sauce	2 tbsp	3	3	0	10
Carb Options Steak Sauce	1 tbsp	1	1	0	5

SAUCES, GRAVIES, AND MARINADES

FOOD	SERVING	TOTAL CARBS (G)	NET CARBS (G)	FIBER (G)	CALORIES
Kraft Barbecue Sauce, CarbWell Original	1 serving (31 g)	3	3	0	15
Steel's Rocky Mountain Barbecue Sauce, Maple Flavor	2 tbsp	10	3	0	40
Steel's Rocky Mountain Barbecue Sauce, Spicy	2 tbsp	2	3	0	15
Steel's Cranberry Sauce	5 tbsp (60 g)	4.5	0	1	20
Steel's Rocky Mountain Hoisin Sauce	2 tbsp (30 g)	2	.25	1	15
Steel's Mango Ginger Chutney	⅓ cup (72 g)	17	16	1	75
Steel's Rocky Mountain Peanut Sauce, Sweet & Spicy	1 tbsp (18 g)	2	0	4.5	34
Steel's Rocky Mountain, Sweet & Sour Sauce	2 tbsp (36 g)	2	0	0	10
Steel's Sugar Free Sweet Ginger Lime Dressing	1 tbsp	1	0	1	68
Walden Farms Honey Barbecue Sauce	2 tbsp	0	0	0	0
Walden Farms Hickory Smoked Barbecue Sauce	2 tbsp	0	0	0	0

SAUCES, GRAVIES, AND MARINADES

FOOD	SERVING	TOTAL CARBS (G)	NET CARBS (G)	FIBER (G)	CALORIES
Walden Farms Original Barbecue Sauce	2 tbsp	0	0	0	0
Walden Farms Thick N Spicy Barbecue Sauce	2 tbsp	0	0	0	0
Walden Farms Seafood Sauce	1 tsp	0	0	0	0
Walden Farms Italian Sun Dried Tomato Marinade	2 tbsp	0	0	0	0
PASTA AND PIZZA SAUCES, BY BRAND					
Bella Vita Low Carb Four Cheese Sauce	½ cup	7	5	2	130
Bella Vita Low Carb Pasta Sauce, Meat Flavored	½ cup	6	4	2	70
Bella Vita Low Carb Pasta Sauce, Roasted Garlic	½ cup	6	4	2	70
Bella Vita Low Carb Pasta Sauce, Tomato Basil	½ cup	6	4	2	70
Keto Pasta Sauce, Marinara	½ cup	6	3	3	60
Keto Pasta Sauce, Meat Flavor	½ cup	7	4	3	70
Keto Pasta Sauce, Vodka Flavor	½ cup	7	4	3	70
Pastalia Low Carb Classic Marinara	½ cup	10	3	7	110

SAUCES, GRAVIES, AND MARINADES

FOOD	SERVING	TOTAL CARBS (G)	NET CARBS (G)	FIBER (G)	CALORIES
Pastalia Low Carb Fra Diavolo	½ cup	10	3	7	110
Pastalia Low Carb Pomodoro Marsala	½ cup	9	6	3	110
Pastalia Low Carb Puttanesca	½ cup	6	5	1	110
Pastalia Low Carb Vodka Sauce	½ cup	4	3	1	110
Pastalia Marinara Sauce	½ cup	10	3	na	60
Walden Farms Alfredo Sauce	¼ cup	0	0	0	0
Walden Farms Bruschetta Sauce	2 tbsp	0	0	0	35
Walden Farms Bruschetta Pesto	1 tbsp	0	0	0	10
Walden Farms Marinara Sauce	⅓ cup	0	0	0	0
Walden Farms Scampi Sauce	2 tbsp	0	0	0	0
GRAVIES					
Au jus, canned	2 tbsp	1	1	0	5
Beef, from jar	2 tbsp	2	2	na	13
Beef, canned	2 tbsp	1	1	t	15
Brown gravy, canned	2 tbsp	2	2	na	12
Chicken, canned	2 tbsp	2	2	t	24
Mushroom, canned	2 tbsp	2	2	t	15
Sausage gravy, ready-to-serve	2 tbsp	2	2	t	48
Turkey, canned	2 tbsp	2	2	t	15

SNACK FOODS (CHIPS, CRACKERS, PRETZELS, POPCORN, AND OTHERS)

FOOD	SERVING	TOTAL CARBS (G)	NET CARBS (G)	FIBER (G)	CALORIES
SAUSAGE, LEAN					
Bratwurst, pork, beef & turkey, light, smoked	2 oz	3	3	0	129
Bratwurst, pork, cooked	1 link	2	2	0	256
Breakfast links, turkey sausage	2 links	1	1	0	129
Hot smoked turkey sausage	2 oz	3	2.5	.5	88
Knockwurst	1 link	2	2	0	221
Meatless sausage	1 link	2	1	1	64
Meatless sausage	1 patty	4	3	1	97
Pork sausage links	2 links	.5	.5	0	165
Pork sausage patties	2 patties	.5	.5	0	199
Pork sausage, Italian	1 link	1	1	0	216
Pork sausage, Polish	1 sausage	4	4	0	740
Pork & beef sausage, cooked	2 links	1	1	0	103
Pork & beef sausage, cooked	2 patties	1.5	1.5	0	214
Smoked sausage, turkey	1 serving	2	2	0	90
Smokies Sausage Little (Pork, Turkey) (Oscar Mayer)	2 links	t	t	0	54
Vienna sausage	7 links	2	2	0	315
SNACK FOODS (CHIPS, CRACKERS, PRETZELS, POPCORN, AND OTHERS)					
CHIPS, GENERIC					
Corn chips, barbecue flavor	¼ bag (7 oz)	28	25	3	259

SNACK FOODS (CHIPS, CRACKERS, PRETZELS, POPCORN, AND OTHERS)

FOOD	SERVING	TOTAL CARBS (G)	NET CARBS (G)	FIBER (G)	CALORIES
Corn chips, plain	¼ bag (7 oz)	28	26	2	267
Potato chips, barbecue flavor	¼ bag (7 oz)	26	24	2	243
Potato chips, cheese flavor	¼ bag (6 oz)	25	23	2	211
Potato chips, made from dried potatoes, plain	¼ can (7 oz)	25	23	2	276
Potato chips, made from dried potatoes, sour cream & onion flavor	¼ can (6.75 oz)	25	24	1	271
Potato chips, plain, made w/partially hydrogenated soybean oil, salted	¼ bag (8 oz)	30	27	3	304
Potato chips, plain, made w/partially hydrogenated soybean oil, unsalted	¼ bag (8 oz)	30	27	3	304
Potato chips, plain, salted	¼ bag (8 oz)	30	27	3	304
Potato chips, plain, unsalted	¼ bag (8 oz)	30	27	3	304
Potato chips, reduced fat	¼ bag (6 oz)	28	25	3	200
Potato chips, sour cream & onion flavor	¼ bag (7 oz)	25	22	3	263
Tortilla chips, taco flavor	¼ bag (8 oz)	36	33	3	272

SNACK FOODS (CHIPS, CRACKERS, PRETZELS, POPCORN, AND OTHERS)

FOOD	SERVING	TOTAL CARBS (G)	NET CARBS (G)	FIBER (G)	CALORIES
CHIPS, BY BRAND					
Atkins Crunchers, BBQ	1 bag (1 oz)	8	4	4	100
Atkins Crunchers, Nacho Cheese	1 bag (1 oz)	8	5	3	100
Atkins Crunchers, Original	1 bag (1 oz)	8	4	4	90
Atkins Crunchers, Sour Cream & Onion	1 bag (1 oz)	8	5	3	100
Carbs-A-Weigh Cheese Chips, Original Flavor	1 oz	0	0	na	55
Carbs-A-Weigh Cheese Chips, BBQ Flavor	1 oz	0	0	na	55
Carb Fit Tortilla Chips, Soy & Corn	1 bag	9	5	4	150
CarbSense Tortilla Chips, Habanero Flavor	15 chips	12	8	4	140
CarbSense Tortilla Chips, Nacho Flavor	15 chips	12	8	4	140
CarbSense Tortilla Chips, Original Flavor	15 chips	12	8	4	145
CarbSense Tortilla Chips, Pico de Gallo Flavor	15 chips	12	8	4	145
Chip's Chips, Cheese Thins, Extra Cheese Flavor	1 bag (1 oz)	0	0	0	140
Chip's Chips, Cheese Thins, Cheddar Flavor	1 bag (1 oz)	0	0	0	140

SNACK FOODS (CHIPS, CRACKERS, PRETZELS, POPCORN, AND OTHERS)

FOOD	SERVING	TOTAL CARBS (G)	NET CARBS (G)	FIBER (G)	CALORIES
Chip's Chips Snackers, BBQ Flavor	1 bag (1 oz)	2	2	0	130
Chip's Chips Snackers, Nacho Flavor	1 bag (1 oz)	2	2	0	130
Chip's Chips Snackers, Sour Cream & Onion Flavor	1 bag (1 oz)	2	2	0	130
Keto Tortilla Chips, Classic Corn	1 oz	8	4	4	150
Keto Tortilla Chips, Cool Ranch	1 oz	8	4	4	150
Keto Tortilla Chips, Nacho Cheese	1 oz	8	4	4	150
CRACKERS, GENERIC					
Butter type	1 serving	10	10	t	79
Cheese, regular	1 cup, bite size	36	34.5	1.5	312
Cheese, sandwich type, w/peanut butter filling	4 crackers	16	15	1	135
Crispbread, rye (including Wasa crispbread)	2 crackers	16	13	3	74
Crispbread, rye, large (triple cracker)	1 cracker	21	17	4	92
Flatbread, Norwegian	3 crackers	14	11	3	63
French onion snack	1 serving	23	22	1	128
Italian ranch snack	1 serving	23	22	1	128
Matzo, plain	1 matzo	23	22	1	111
Matzo, whole wheat	1 matzo	22	19	3	98
Melba toast, rye	4 toasts	15	13	2	76
Melba toast, wheat	4 toasts	15	13	2	76

SNACK FOODS (CHIPS, CRACKERS, PRETZELS, POPCORN, AND OTHERS)

FOOD	SERVING	TOTAL CARBS (G)	NET CARBS (G)	FIBER (G)	CALORIES
Oyster	½ cup	16	15	1	98
Oyster, low salt	½ cup	16	15	1	98
Salsa snack	1 serving	23	22	1	128
Rye, sandwich type, w/peanut butter filling	4 crackers	17	16	1	135
Rye wafers, plain	2 wafers	18	13	5	74
Rye wafers, seasoned, large (triple cracker)	1 wafer	16	11	5	84
Saltines	1 serving	10	10	t	59
Snack type, sandwich type w/cheese filling	4 crackers	17	16.5	.5	134
Wheat, sandwich type, w/cheese filling	4 crackers	16	15	1	139
Wheat, sandwich type, w/peanut butter filling	4 crackers	15	14	1	139
Wheat, thin type	1 serving	20	19	1	136
Whole wheat crackers	4 crackers	10	8	2	72
CRACKERS, BY BRAND					
Andre's Carbosave Cheddar Cheese Crackerbread	1 oz	3	2	1	90
Andre's Carbosave Sweet Cinnamon Crackerbread	1 oz	3	2	1	90
Andre's Carbosave Roasted Garlic Crackerbread	1 oz	3	2	1	90
Andre's Carbosave Crackerbread, Mild Chili	1 oz	8	4	4	140

SNACK FOODS (CHIPS, CRACKERS, PRETZELS, POPCORN, AND OTHERS)

FOOD	SERVING	TOTAL CARBS (G)	NET CARBS (G)	FIBER (G)	CALORIES
Andre's Carbosave Original Crackerbread	1 oz	3	2	1	90
Andre's Carbosave Old World Country Onion Crackerbread	1 oz	3	2	1	90
Andre's Carbosave Old World Rye Crackerbread	1 oz	3	2	1	90
Andre's Carbosave Zesty Italian Crackerbread	1 oz	3	2	1	90
Atkins Flatbread Crackers, Cheddar	3 crackers	8	4	4	140
Atkins Flatbread Crackers, Country Onion	3 crackers	8	4	4	140
Atkins Flatbread Crackers, Garlic	3 crackers	8	4	4	140
Atkins Flatbread Crackers, Old World Rye	3 crackers	8	4	4	140
Atkins Flatbread Crackers, Parmesan	3 crackers	8	4	4	140
Atkins Flatbread Crackers, Plain	3 crackers	8	4	4	140
Atkins Flatbread Crackers, Toasted Sesame	3 crackers	8	4	4	140
Atkins Flatbread Crackers, Zesty Italian	3 crackers	8	4	4	140

SNACK FOODS (CHIPS, CRACKERS, PRETZELS, POPCORN, AND OTHERS)

FOOD	SERVING	TOTAL CARBS (G)	NET CARBS (G)	FIBER (G)	CALORIES
Atkins Whole Wheat Crackers	2 crackers	5	5	0	50
Atkins Sesame Crackers	2 crackers	5	5	0	50
Blue Diamond Nut Thins, Almond	16 crackers	20	20	t	120
Blue Diamond Nut Thins, Hazelnut	16 crackers	21	21	t	120
Blue Diamond Nut Thins, Pecan	16 crackers	21	21	0	120
Blue Diamond Nut Thins, Smokehouse Almond	16 crackers	20	20	t	120
Cheeters Crackers, Garlic	3 crackers	6	1	5	140
Cheeters Crackers, Onion	3 crackers	6	1	5	140
Cheeters Crackers, Plain	3 crackers	6	1	5	140
Cheeters Crackers, Rye	3 crackers	6	1	5	140
Cheeters Crackers, Sesame	3 crackers	6	1	5	140
Cheeters Crackers, Sweet Cinnamon	3 crackers	6	1	5	140
Heavenly Desserts Crackers, Sesame	1 cracker	2.5	2.5	0	16
Heavenly Desserts Crackers, White Wheat	1 cracker	2.5	2.5	0	16

SNACK FOODS (CHIPS, CRACKERS, PRETZELS, POPCORN, AND OTHERS)

FOOD	SERVING	TOTAL CARBS (G)	NET CARBS (G)	FIBER (G)	CALORIES
MiniCarb Soy Thins Original	16 crackers	8	5	3	120
No-Carb Kitchen Gourmet Cheese Crackers, Aged Parmesan	3 crackers	0	0	0	75
No-Carb Kitchen Gourmet Cheese Crackers, Caraway	3 crackers	t	0	t	75
No-Carb Kitchen Gourmet Cheese Crackers, Onion Poppyseed	3 crackers	t	0	t	75
No-Carb Kitchen Gourmet Cheese Crackers, Sesame	3 crackers	t	0	t	75
POPCORN					
Popcorn, caramel, coated, w/peanuts	⅔ cup	23	22	1	113
Popcorn, caramel, coated, w/o peanuts	⅔ cup	22	20.5	1.5	122
Popcorn, cheese flavor	2 cups	11	9	2	116
Popcorn, oil popped	2 cups	13	11	2	110
PRETZELS, GENERIC					
Cheddar cheese pretzels	10 pieces	20	20	na	139
Chocolate-coated pretzel	1 pretzel	8	8	na	50
Plain pretzels, hard	10 twists	48	46	2	229
Pretzel, soft	1 large (143 g)	99	97	2	483

SNACK FOODS (CHIPS, CRACKERS, PRETZELS, POPCORN, AND OTHERS)

FOOD	SERVING	TOTAL CARBS (G)	NET CARBS (G)	FIBER (G)	CALORIES
Whole wheat pretzels, hard	2 oz	46	42	4	206
PRETZELS, BY BRAND					
CarbSense Soy Pretzels	15 pretzels	12	8	4	100
Pure De-lite Chocolate Pretzels, Dark Chocolate	1 oz	14	4	2	140
Pure De-lite Chocolate Pretzels, White Chocolate	1 oz	14	4	2	140
Pure De-lite Chocolate Pretzels, Chocolate	1 oz	14	4	2	140
OTHER SNACKS, GENERIC					
Banana chips	1 oz	16	14	2	147
Beef jerky, chopped & formed	1 oz	3	2	1	116
Beef sticks, smoked	1 oz	2	2	0	155
Cheese puffs or twists	1 oz	15	15	0	156
Cheese puffs or twists, low fat	1 oz	20	17	3	122
Corn, air-popped popcorn	2 cups	12	10	2	61
Corn nuts, barbecue flavor	1 oz	20	18	2	123
Corn nuts, nacho flavor	1 oz	20	18	2	124
Corn nuts, plain	1 oz	20	18	2	126
Pork skins, barbecue flavor	1 oz	0	0	0	152
Pork skins, plain	1 oz	0	0	0	154
Potato sticks	1 oz	15	14	1	147

SNACK FOODS (CHIPS, CRACKERS, PRETZELS, POPCORN, AND OTHERS)

FOOD	SERVING	TOTAL CARBS (G)	NET CARBS (G)	FIBER (G)	CALORIES
Sesame sticks, wheat based, salted	1 oz	13	12	1	153
Snack mix, original flavor	1 cup	37	33	4	260
OTHER SNACKS, BY BRAND					
Atkins Just The Cheese Rounds, White Cheddar, Low Salt	1 serving (1 oz)	1	t	0	160
Atkins Energy Burst Protein Snack Mix	1 bag (30 g)	7	5	2	140
Carb Fit Twirls, Cool Ranch Crispy Soy Snacks	1 bag	8	5	3	110
Carb Fit Twirls, Nacho Cheese Crispy Soy Snacks	1 bag	8	5	3	120
Carb Slim Bites, Chocolate Caramel	28 g	14	0	6	118
Carb Slim Bites, Peanut Butter	28 g	14	0	6	118
Chex Mix (General Mills)	1 oz (approx. ⅔ cup)	18	16	2	120
Doctor's CarbRite Diet Brown Rice Cake, Dark Chocolate	1 cake (35 g)	24	9	3	152
Doctor's CarbRite Diet Brown Rice Cake, Milk Chocolate	1 cake (35 g)	22	9	1	150
Geraldine's Bodacious Cheese Straws	12 pieces	6	4	2	160
Getmor Soy Snacks, Herb & Garlic	1 oz	7	3	4	121

SNACK FOODS (CHIPS, CRACKERS, PRETZELS, POPCORN, AND OTHERS)

FOOD	SERVING	TOTAL CARBS (G)	NET CARBS (G)	FIBER (G)	CALORIES
Getmor Soy Snacks, Jalapeño & Cheese	1 oz	7	3	4	118
Getmor Soy Snacks, Tamari Sauce Flavor	1 oz	5	2	3	102
Gram's Gourmet Flax 'n Nut Crunchies, Cinnamon Toast	⅓ cup	6.7	2.7	4	234
Gram's Gourmet Flax 'n Nut Crunchies, Vanilla Almond Crunch	⅓ cup	6.7	2.7	4	234
Gram's Gourmet Cheddar Cheese Crunchies	½ oz	2	2	0	80
Gram's Gourmet Sweet Cinnamon & Butter Crunchies	½ oz	0	0	0	70
Jack Link's Beef Jerky, Original	1 oz	3	3	0	80
Jack Link's Beef Jerky, Peppered	1 oz	4	4	0	80
Jack Link's Beef Jerky, Teriyaki	1 oz	5	5	0	80
Jack Link's Beef Jerky, Sweet & Hot	1 oz	5	5	0	80
Jack Link's Turkey Jerky, Original	1 oz	3	3	0	80
Just The Cheese Snacks, Crunchy Bacon Cheese	1 serving (1 oz)	1	1	0	150

328 SNACK FOODS (CHIPS, CRACKERS, PRETZELS, POPCORN, AND OTHERS)

FOOD	SERVING	TOTAL CARBS (G)	NET CARBS (G)	FIBER (G)	CALORIES
Just The Cheese Snacks, Cheddar Cheese, Low Salt	1 serving (1 oz)	1	1	0	150
Just The Cheese Snacks, Cool Ranch Cheese	1 serving (1 oz)	1	1	0	150
Just The Cheese Snacks, Herb & Garlic Cheese	1 serving (1 oz)	1	1	0	150
Just The Cheese Snacks, Honey Dijon Cheese	1 serving (1 oz)	1	1	0	150
Just The Cheese Snacks, Jalapeño Cheese	1 serving (1 oz)	1	1	0	150
Just The Cheese Snacks, Nacho Cheese	1 serving (1 oz)	1	1	0	150
Just The Cheese Snacks, Pizza Flavor Cheese	1 serving (1 oz)	1	1	0	150
Just The Cheese Snacks, Sour Cream & Onion	1 serving (1 oz)	1	1	0	160
Just The Cheese Snacks, White Cheddar	1 serving (1 oz)	1	1	0	150
King B Beef Steak, Original Beef Jerky	1 oz	3	3	0	70

SNACK FOODS (CHIPS, CRACKERS, PRETZELS, POPCORN, AND OTHERS)

FOOD	SERVING	TOTAL CARBS (G)	NET CARBS (G)	FIBER (G)	CALORIES
King B Beef Steak, Peppered Beef Jerky	1 oz	3	3	0	70
King B Beef Steak, Teriyaki Beef Jerky	1 oz	5	5	0	80
Lean Protein Bites, Milk Chocolate	1 serving (1 oz)	1	1	0	120
Lean Protein Bites, Peanut Butter	1 serving (1 oz)	1	1	0	120
Lean Protein Bites, White Chocolate	1 serving (1 oz)	2	1	0	120
Ostrim Meat Stick, Barbecue Flavor Ostrich & Beef Snack	1 stick (42 g)	3	2	1	80
Ostrim Meat Stick, Natural Flavor Ostrich & Beef Snack	1 stick (42 g)	4	4	na	90
Ostrim Meat Stick, Pepper Flavor Ostrich & Beef Snack	1 stick (42 g)	1	1	na	80
Ostrim Meat Stick, Teriyaki Flavor Ostrich & Beef Snack	1 stick (42 g)	3	3	na	80
Pumpkorn, Caramel Flavor Pumpkin Seeds	⅓ cup	4	2	2	150
Pumpkorn, Chili Flavor Pumpkin Seeds	⅓ cup	4	2	2	150

330 SOFT DRINKS

FOOD	SERVING	TOTAL CARBS (G)	NET CARBS (G)	FIBER (G)	CALORIES
Pumpkorn, Curry Flavor Pumpkin Seeds	⅓ cup	4	2	2	150
Pumpkorn, Maple Vanilla Flavor Pumpkin Seeds	⅓ cup	4	2	2	150
Pumpkorn, Mildly Original Flavor Pumpkin Seeds	⅓ cup	4	2	2	150
Pumpkorn, Mesquite Flavor Pumpkin Seeds	⅓ cup	4	2	2	150
Pumpkorn, Original Flavor Pumpkin Seeds	⅓ cup	4	2	2	150
Robert's American Gourmet, Girlfriend's Booty Crunchy Snack Mix, Plain Flavor	1 oz	8	5	3	120
Robert's American Gourmet, Girlfriend's Booty Crunchy Snack Mix, Barbecue Flavor	1 oz	8	5	3	120
Soy Nutty Crunchies	1 serving (22 g)	8	2	6	97
SOFT DRINKS					
Birch Beer, Diet (Boylon's)	1 bottle	0	0	0	0
Carbonated/mineral water	1 cup	0	0	0	0
Chocolate flavor soda	1 can or bottle (12 fl oz)	39	39	0	155

SOFT DRINKS

FOOD	SERVING	TOTAL CARBS (G)	NET CARBS (G)	FIBER (G)	CALORIES
Club soda	1 can (12 fl oz)	0	0	0	0
Cola, w/caffeine	1 can or bottle (12 fl oz)	40	40	0	155
Cola, w/higher caffeine	1 can or bottle (12 fl oz)	40	40	0	155
Cola, w/o caffeine	1 can or bottle (12 fl oz)	40	40	0	155
Cola, w/o caffeine, supersized, large	1 drink (32 fl oz)	106	106	0	413
Cola, w/o caffeine, supersized, extra large	1 drink (44 fl oz)	145	145	0	568
Coca-Cola C2, Lower Sugar Cola (Coca-Cola)	1 drink (8 oz)	12	12	0	45
Diet soft drinks	1 can (12 fl oz)	t	t	0	4
Cream soda	1 can or bottle (12 fl oz)	50	50	0	189
Ginger ale	1 can or bottle (12 fl oz)	32	32	0	124
Grape soda	1 can or bottle (12 fl oz)	42	42	0	160
Lemonade, low calorie, w/aspartame, prepared	1 cup	1	1	0	5
Lemonade, Sugar Free, Instant (Atkins)	½ tsp for 8 oz drink	1	1	0	8
Lemonade, No Sugar Added (Calypso)	1 bottle (8 fl oz)	3	3	0	12
Lemon-lime soda, w/o caffeine	1 can or bottle (12 fl oz)	38	38	0	147

SOUPS

FOOD	SERVING	TOTAL CARBS (G)	NET CARBS (G)	FIBER (G)	CALORIES
Lemon-lime soda, w/caffeine	1 can or bottle (12 fl oz)	38	38	0	147
Orange soda	1 can or bottle (12 fl oz)	46	46	0	179
Pepper type, w/caffeine	1 can or bottle (12 fl oz)	38	38	0	151
Root beer	1 can or bottle (12 fl oz)	40	40	0	152
Root Beer, Diet (Boylon's)	1 bottle	0	0	0	0
Root Beer (Root 66)	1 bottle (8 oz)	0	0	0	0
Soft drink mix, tropical flavor, unsweetened, powder	1 serving	t	t	0	1
Strawberry Lemonade, No Sugar Added (Calypso)	1 bottle (8 fl oz)	3	3	0	12

SOUPS

SOUP, INSTANT, BY BRAND

FOOD	SERVING	TOTAL CARBS (G)	NET CARBS (G)	FIBER (G)	CALORIES
AlpineAire Bay Shrimp Bisque, Low Carb Soup Mix	1 container	7	6	1	70
AlpineAire Beefy Vegetable, Low Carb Soup Mix	1 container	5	4	1	70
AlpineAire Broccoli Cheddar, Low Carb Soup Mix	1 container	6	5	1	70
AlpineAire Chicken w/ Asparagus, Low Carb Soup Mix	1 container	5	4	1	130

FOOD	SERVING	TOTAL CARBS (G)	NET CARBS (G)	FIBER (G)	CALORIES
AlpineAire Chicken Vegetable, Low Carb Soup Mix	1 container	5	3	2	90
AlpineAire Mushroom Chicken, Low Carb Soup Mix	1 container	6	4	2	70
Atkins Bay Shrimp Bisque Soup Mix	10 oz cup	6	5	1	150
Atkins Beefy Vegetable Soup Mix	10 oz cup	5	4	1	70
Atkins Broccoli & Cheese Soup Mix	10 oz cup	3	1	2	78
Atkins Broccoli w/Cheddar Cheese Soup Mix	10 oz cup	6	4	2	140
Atkins Chicken/Cheese Enchilada Soup Mix	10 oz cup	4	2	2	94
Atkins Chicken Noodle Soup Mix	10 oz cup	3	2	1	40
Atkins Cream of Mushroom Soup Mix	10 oz cup	2	2	0	51
Atkins Mushroom & Chicken w/Roasted Garlic Soup Mix	10 oz cup	7	6	1	130
Carb'Tastic Asian Ginger Broccoli Soup Mix	1 pkt	11	2	9	80
Carb'Tastic Broccoli Cheddar Soup Mix	1 pkt	13	6	7	110
Carb'Tastic Hot & Sour Soup Mix	1 pkt	7	6	1	70

334 SOUPS

FOOD	SERVING	TOTAL CARBS (G)	NET CARBS (G)	FIBER (G)	CALORIES
Carb'Tastic Shiitake Mushroom Soup Mix	1 pkt	7	6	1	80
Carb'Tastic Sundried Tomato Basil Soup Mix	1 pkt	10	3	7	70
Carb'Tastic Vegetarian Beef w/Barley Soup Mix	1 pkt	10	6	4	70
Carb'Tastic Vegetarian Chicken Gumbo Soup Mix	1 pkt	9	5	4	90
Carb'Tastic Vegetarian Mandarin Chicken Soup Mix	1 pkt	13	3	10	90
Dixie Diners' Club Broccoli & Cheese Soup Mix	1 cup (16.7 g)	3	2	1	78
Dixie Diners' Club Chicken & Cheese Enchilada Soup Mix	1 cup (18 g)	4	2	2	94
Dixie Diners' Club Chicken Noodle Soup Mix	1 cup (11 g)	3	2	1	40
LC Homestyles Beef Chili Soup Mix	1 cup (227 g)	13	5	8	280
LC Homestyles Chicken Chili Soup Mix	1 cup (227 g)	13	3	10	190
LC Homestyles Steak Chili Soup Mix	1 cup (227 g)	14	5	9	260
MiniCarb Soup Mix, Miso	1 cup (20.9 g dry)	5	4	1	33

FOOD	SERVING	TOTAL CARBS (G)	NET CARBS (G)	FIBER (G)	CALORIES
MiniCarb Soup Mix, Szechuan Beef	1 cup (20.9 g dry)	4	2	0	24
MiniCarb Soup Mix, Thai Coconut Cream	1 cup (20.9 g dry)	9	4	1	100
SOUPS, GENERIC					
Bean w/frankfurters, canned, prepared w/water	1 cup	22	22	na	188
Bean w/ham, chunky, ready-to-serve	1 cup	27	16	11	231
Bean w/pork, canned, prepared w/water	1 cup	23	14	9	172
Beef broth or bouillon, canned, ready-to-serve	1 cup	t	t	0	17
Beef broth or bouillon, powder, prepared w/water	1 cup	2	2	0	20
Beef broth, cube, prepared w/water	1 cup	1	1	0	7
Beef w/country vegetables, chunky, ready-to-serve	1 serving	16	16	0	153
Beef, chunky, ready-to-serve	1 cup	20	19	1	170
Beef mushroom, canned, prepared w/water	1 cup	6	6	t	73
Beef noodle, canned, prepared w/water	1 cup	9	9	t	83

336 SOUPS

FOOD	SERVING	TOTAL CARBS (G)	NET CARBS (G)	FIBER (G)	CALORIES
Beef noodle, dehydrated, prepared w/water	1 pkt	4	3	1	30
Black bean, canned, prepared w/water	1 cup	20	15	5	116
Cauliflower, dehydrated, prepared w/water	1 cup	11	11	na	69
Cheese, canned, prepared w/milk	1 cup	16	15	1	231
Cheese, canned, prepared w/water	1 cup	11	10	1	156
Chicken broth, canned, prepared w/water	1 cup	1	1	0	39
Chicken broth, cube, prepared w/water	1 cup	2	2	na	12
Chicken broth or bouillon, dehydrated, prepared w/water	1 pkt	1	1	0	16
Chicken corn chowder, chunky, ready-to-serve	1 serving	18	16	2	238
Chicken gumbo, canned, prepared w/water	1 cup	8	6	2	56
Chicken w/dumplings, canned, prepared w/water	1 cup	6	5.5	.5	96
Chicken, mushroom chowder, chunky, ready-to-serve	1 serving	17	14	3	192
Chicken, mushroom, canned, prepared w/water	1 cup	9	9	t	132

SOUPS

FOOD	SERVING	TOTAL CARBS (G)	NET CARBS (G)	FIBER (G)	CALORIES
Chicken, chunky, ready-to-serve	1 cup	17	15	2	178
Chicken noodle, canned, prepared w/water	1 cup	9	8	1	75
Chicken noodle, chunky, ready-to-serve	1 serving	14	14	na	114
Chicken noodle, dehydrated, prepared w/water	1 cup	7	7	t	43
Chicken noodle w/ celery & onions, ready-to-serve	1 serving	9	9	na	95
Chicken vegetable, canned, prepared w/water	1 cup	9	8	1	75
Chicken vegetable, chunky, reduced fat, reduced sodium, ready-to-serve	1 serving	15	15	na	96
Chicken vegetable, dehydrated, prepared w/water	1 cup	8	8	na	50
Chicken w/rice, canned, prepared w/water	1 cup	7	6	1	60
Clam chowder, Manhattan style, canned, prepared w/water	1 cup	12	10.5	1.5	78
Clam chowder, Manhattan style, chunky, ready-to-serve	1 cup	19	16	3	134

SOUPS

FOOD	SERVING	TOTAL CARBS (G)	NET CARBS (G)	FIBER (G)	CALORIES
Clam chowder, New England, canned, prepared w/milk	1 cup	17	15	2	164
Clam chowder, New England style, canned, prepared w/water	1 cup	12	10.5	1.5	95
Consomme, canned, prepared w/water	1 cup	2	2	0	29
Cream of asparagus, canned, prepared w/milk	1 cup	16	15	1	161
Cream of celery, canned, prepared w/milk	1 cup	15	14	1	164
Cream of chicken, canned, prepared w/milk	1 cup	15	15	t	191
Cream of mushroom, canned, prepared w/milk	1 cup	15	14.5	.5	203
Crab soup, ready-to-serve	1 cup	10	9	1	76
Cream of asparagus, dehydrated, prepared w/water	1 cup	9	9	na	58
Cream of celery, dehydrated, prepared w/water	1 cup	10	10	na	64
Cream of mushroom, canned, prepared w/water	1 cup	9	8.5	.5	129

FOOD	SERVING	TOTAL CARBS (G)	NET CARBS (G)	FIBER (G)	CALORIES
Cream of onion, canned, prepared w/milk	1 cup	18	17	1	186
Cream of onion, canned, prepared w/water	1 cup	13	12	1	107
Cream of potato, canned, prepared w/milk	1 cup	17	16.5	.5	149
Cream of potato, canned, prepared w/water	1 cup	11	10.5	.5	73
Cream of shrimp, canned, prepared w/milk	1 cup	14	14	t	164
Cream of shrimp, canned, prepared w/water	1 cup	8	8	t	90
Cream of vegetable, dehydrated, prepared w/water	1 cup	12	11.5	.5	107
Gazpacho, ready-to-serve	1 cup	4	3.5	.5	46
Leek soup, dehydrated, prepared w/water	1 cup	11	8	3	71
Lentil soup, ready-to-serve	1 cup	20	14	6	126
Minestrone, chunky, ready-to-serve	1 cup	21	15	6	127
Minestrone, canned, prepared w/water	1 cup	11	10	1	82

SOUPS

FOOD	SERVING	TOTAL CARBS (G)	NET CARBS (G)	FIBER (G)	CALORIES
Minestrone, dehydrated, prepared w/water	1 cup	12	12	na	79
Mushroom, dehydrated, prepared w/water	1 pkt	9	8	1	74
Mushroom barley, canned, prepared w/water	1 cup	12	11	1	73
Mushroom w/beef stock, canned, prepared w/water	1 cup	9	8	1	85
Onion, canned, prepared w/water	1 cup	8	7	1	58
Onion, dehydrated, prepared w/water	1 cup	5	4	1	27
Oyster stew, canned, prepared w/milk	1 cup	10	10	0	135
Oyster stew, canned, prepared w/water	1 cup	4	4	na	58
Pea, green, canned, prepared w/milk	1 cup	32	29	3	239
Pea soup, canned, prepared w/water	1 cup	27	23	3	165
Pea soup, dehydrated, prepared w/water	1 cup	17	15	2	101
Potato ham chowder, chunky, ready-to-serve	1 serving	13	12	1	192
Sirloin burger w/ vegetables, ready-to-serve	1 serving	16	10	6	185
Split pea, ready-to-serve	1 cup	30	25	5	180

FOOD	SERVING	TOTAL CARBS (G)	NET CARBS (G)	FIBER (G)	CALORIES
Split pea w/ham, chunky, ready-to-serve	1 cup	27	23	4	185
Split pea w/ham, canned, prepared w/water	1 cup	28	26	2	190
Split pea w/ham, chunky, reduced fat, reduced sodium, ready-to-serve	1 serving	27	27	na	185
Tomato beef w/noodle, canned, prepared w/water	1 cup	21	20	1	139
Tomato bisque, canned, prepared w/milk	1 cup	29	28.5	.5	198
Tomato bisque, canned, prepared w/water	1 cup	24	23.5	.5	124
Tomato, canned, prepared w/milk	1 cup	22	19	3	161
Tomato, canned, prepared w/water	1 cup	17	16.5	.5	85
Tomato, dehydrated, prepared w/water	1 pkt	15	15	t	78
Tomato rice, canned, prepared w/water	1 cup	22	20.5	1.5	119
Tomato vegetable, dehydrated, prepared w/water	1 pkt	8	8	t	42
Turkey, chunky, ready-to-serve	1 cup	14	14	na	135
Turkey noodle, canned, prepared w/water	1 cup	9	8	1	68

342 SOY AND VEGETARIAN FOODS

FOOD	SERVING	TOTAL CARBS (G)	NET CARBS (G)	FIBER (G)	CALORIES
Turkey vegetable, canned, prepared w/water	1 cup	9	8.5	.5	72
Vegetable, chunky ready-to-serve	1 cup	19	18	1	122
Vegetable beef, canned, prepared w/water	1 cup	10	9.5	.5	78
Vegetable beef, dehydrated, prepared w/water	1 cup	8	7.5	.5	53
Vegetable beef, microwaveable, ready-to-serve	1 serving	10	6	4	128
Vegetable w/beef broth, canned, prepared w/water	1 cup	13	12.5	.5	82
Vegetarian vegetable, canned, prepared w/water	1 cup	12	11.5	.5	72

SOY AND VEGETARIAN FOODS

FOOD	SERVING	TOTAL CARBS (G)	NET CARBS (G)	FIBER (G)	CALORIES
Black bean burger	1 patty (2.7 oz)	16	11	5	110
Hotdog, meatless	1 link	2	0	2	118
Soybeans, boiled, w/salt	½ cup	9	4	5	149
Soybeans, boiled, w/o salt	½ cup	9	4	5	149
Soybeans, dry roasted	2 tbsp	7	5	2	101
Soy burger	1 patty	9	9	na	110
Soy cheese, swiss	2 slices (0.7 oz)	1	1	na	120
Soy cheese, mozzarella	2 slices (1 oz)	2	2	na	120

FOOD	SERVING	TOTAL CARBS (G)	NET CARBS (G)	FIBER (G)	CALORIES
Soy cheese, cheddar	2 slices (0.7 oz)	1	1	na	120
Soy cheese, American	2 slices (0.7 oz)	1	1	na	120
Soy milk, plain	1 cup	4	1	3	81
Soy pasta	1 serving (2 oz or 1/6 box)	34	33	1	200
Tempeh	½ cup	8	8	na	160
Tofu, silken, extra firm	1 slice	2	2	na	46
Tofu, silken, firm	1 slice	2	2	na	52
Tofu, silken, light extra firm	1 slice	1	1	0	32
Tofu, silken, soft	1 slice	2	2	na	46
Tofu, silken, light firm	1 slice	1	1	0	31
Vegetable burger	1 patty	7	1	6	138

VEAL

VEAL

FOOD	SERVING	TOTAL CARBS (G)	NET CARBS (G)	FIBER (G)	CALORIES
Breast, point half, lean & fat, boneless, braised	4 oz	0	0	0	281
Breast, whole, boneless, lean & fat, braised	4 oz	0	0	0	301
Retail cuts, lean & fat, cooked	4 oz	0	0	0	262
Breast, whole, lean only, boneless, braised	4 oz	0	0	0	247
Cubed for stewing, lean only, braised	4 oz	0	0	0	213
Ground, broiled	4 oz	0	0	0	195
Leg, top round, lean only, braised	4 oz	0	0	0	230

344 VEAL

FOOD	SERVING	TOTAL CARBS (G)	NET CARBS (G)	FIBER (G)	CALORIES
Leg, top round, lean only, pan fried	4 oz	0	0	0	207
Leg, top round, lean only, roasted	4 oz	0	0	0	170
Loin, braised	4 oz	0	0	0	156
Rib, braised	4 oz	0	0	0	247
Rib, roasted	4 oz	0	0	0	201
Shank, lean only, braised	4 oz	0	0	0	201
Shoulder, arm, braised	4 oz	0	0	0	228
Shoulder, arm, lean only roasted	4 oz	0	0	0	186
Shoulder, blade, lean only, braised	4 oz	0	0	0	224
Shoulder, blade, lean only, roasted	4 oz	0	0	0	194
Shoulder, whole (arm & shoulder), lean only braised	4 oz	0	0	0	226
Shoulder, whole (arm & shoulder), lean only, roasted	4 oz	0	0	0	193
Sirloin, lean only, braised	4 oz	0	0	0	231
Sirloin, lean only, roasted	4 oz	0	0	0	190
VEAL VARIETY MEATS, LEAN					
Veal liver, braised	4 oz	3	3	0	187
Veal spleen, braised	4 oz	0	0	0	146

VEGETABLES AND VEGETABLE JUICES

VEGETABLES

FOOD	SERVING	TOTAL CARBS (G)	NET CARBS (G)	FIBER (G)	CALORIES
Alfalfa sprouts, raw	1 cup	1	0	1	10
Artichoke, hearts, canned in water	4 oz	8	7	1	42
Artichoke hearts, boiled, drained	½ cup	9	4	5	42
Artichoke, whole, globe or French boiled, drained	1 medium	13	6	7	60
Arugula, raw, chopped	1 cup	1	1	t	6
Asparagus, canned, drained	½ cup	3	1	2	23
Asparagus, from fresh, cuts & tips, cooked	½ cup	4	3	1	22
Asparagus, from fresh, spears, boiled & drained, w/salt	6 spears	4	2	2	22
Asparagus, from fresh, spears, boiled & drained, w/o salt	6 spears	4	3	1	22
Asparagus, from frozen, spears, boiled, drained	6 spears	4	3	1	25
Bamboo shoots, canned, drained slices	½ cup	1	0	1	7
Bamboo shoots, canned, drained slices	½ cup	2	1	1	12
Bamboo shoots, raw, pieces	1 cup	8	5	3	41
Beans, snap, green, canned	½ cup	3	2	1	14

VEGETABLES AND VEGETABLE JUICES

FOOD	SERVING	TOTAL CARBS (G)	NET CARBS (G)	FIBER (G)	CALORIES
Beans, snap, green, from fresh, boiled	½ cup	5	3	2	22
Beans, snap, green, from frozen, boiled	½ cup	4	2	2	19
Beans, snap, green, raw	1 cup	8	4	4	34
Beans, snap, yellow, canned	½ cup	3	2	1	14
Beans, snap, yellow, from fresh, boiled	½ cup	5	3	2	22
Beans, snap, yellow, from frozen, boiled	½ cup	4	2	2	19
Beans, snap, yellow, raw	1 cup	8	4	4	34
Beets, raw	1 cup	13	9	4	58
Beets, raw (2" dia)	2 beets	16	11	5	71
Beets, canned, diced, drained	½ cup	6	5	1	24
Beets, canned, shredded, drained	½ cup	7	5	2	30
Beets, canned, sliced, drained	½ cup	6	5	1	26
Beets, canned, whole, drained	½ cup	6	5	1	25
Beets, canned, drained	2 beets	3	2	1	15
Beets, from fresh, sliced, boiled, drained	½ cup	8	6	2	37
Beets, canned, pickled, slices	½ cup	18	15	3	74
Beets, whole, from fresh, cooked	2 beets	10	8	2	44
Beets, Harvard, canned, slices	½ cup	22	19	3	90

VEGETABLES AND VEGETABLE JUICES 347

FOOD	SERVING	TOTAL CARBS (G)	NET CARBS (G)	FIBER (G)	CALORIES
Beet greens, boiled, drained	½ cup	4	2	2	19
Beet greens, raw, chopped	1 cup	2	1	1	7
Broccoli, Chinese, cooked	½ cup	2	1	1	10
Broccoli, boiled, drained	1 large stalk (11"–12" long)	14	6	8	78
Broccoli, boiled, drained	1 medium stalk (7½"–8" long)	9	4	5	50
Broccoli, boiled, drained	1 small stalk (5" long)	7	3	4	39
Broccoli, chopped, boiled, drained	½ cup	4	2	2	22
Broccoli florets, raw	1 cup	4	4	na	20
Broccoli, frozen, chopped, boiled, drained	½ cup	5	2	3	26
Broccoli in cheese flavored sauce, frozen	1 cup	15	15	0	113
Broccoli, frozen, spears, boiled, drained	½ cup	5	2	3	26
Broccoli, raw, chopped	1 cup	5	2	3	25
Broccoli, raw, spears	2 spears	3	1	2	17
Broccoli, raw, stalk	1 stalk	8	3.5	4.5	42
Brussels sprouts, boiled, drained	6 sprouts	11	8	3	49

VEGETABLES AND VEGETABLE JUICES

FOOD	SERVING	TOTAL CARBS (G)	NET CARBS (G)	FIBER (G)	CALORIES
Brussels sprouts, boiled, drained	½ cup	7	5	2	30
Brussels sprouts, frozen, boiled, drained	½ cup	6	3	3	33
Brussels sprouts, raw	1 cup	8	5	3	38
Brussels sprouts, raw	6 sprouts	10	6	4	49
Butternut squash, cubes, baked	½ cup	11	11	na	41
Butternut squash, frozen, boiled	½ cup	12	12	na	47
Cabbage, Chinese (bok choy), shredded, boiled, drained	½ cup	2	1	1	10
Cabbage, Chinese (bok choy), shredded, raw	1 cup	2	1	1	9
Cabbage, Chinese (*pe tsai*), shredded, boiled, drained	½ cup	1	0	1	8
Cabbage, Chinese (*pe tsai*), shredded, raw	1 cup	2	1	2	12
Cabbage, raw, chopped	1 cup	5	3	2	22
Cabbage, raw, shredded	1 cup	4	2	2	18
Cabbage, shredded, boiled, drained	½ cup	3	1	2	17
Cabbage, napa, cooked	½ cup	1	1	na	7
Cabbage, red, shredded, boiled, drained	½ cup	3	1.5	1.5	16

VEGETABLES AND VEGETABLE JUICES 349

FOOD	SERVING	TOTAL CARBS (G)	NET CARBS (G)	FIBER (G)	CALORIES
Cabbage, red, raw, chopped	1 cup	5	3	2	24
Cabbage, red, raw, shredded	1 cup	4	3	1	19
Cabbage, savoy, raw, shredded	1 cup	4	2	2	19
Cabbage, savoy, shredded, boiled, drained	½ cup	4	2	2	17
Carrots, baby, large, raw	6 carrots	7	5	2	34
Carrots, baby, medium, raw	6 carrots	5	4	1	23
Carrots, canned, mashed	½ cup	6	4	2	29
Carrots, canned, sliced	½ cup	4	3	1	18
Carrots, raw, chopped	1 cup	13	9	4	55
Carrots, raw, grated	1 cup	11	8	3	47
Carrots, raw, sliced	1 cup	12	8	4	52
Carrots, sliced, boiled, drained	½ cup	8	5	3	35
Carrots, frozen, sliced, boiled	½ cup	6	3	3	26
Cauliflower, raw	1 cup	5	2.5	2.5	25
Cauliflower, raw, florets	6 florets	4	2	2	20
Cauliflower, boiled, drained	½ cup	3	1	2	14
Cauliflower, florets, boiled, drained	6 pieces	4	1	3	25

VEGETABLES AND VEGETABLE JUICES

FOOD	SERVING	TOTAL CARBS (G)	NET CARBS (G)	FIBER (G)	CALORIES
Cauliflower, frozen, boiled, drained	½ cup	3	1	2	17
Cauliflower, green, cooked	¼ head	6	3	3	29
Cauliflower, green, raw	1 cup	4	2	2	20
Cauliflower, green, florets	6 florets	9	4	5	47
Celery, diced, boiled, drained	½ cup	3	2	1	14
Celery, diced, raw	1 cup	4	2	2	19
Celery, strips, raw	1 cup	5	3	2	20
Chard, swiss, chopped, boiled, drained	½ cup	4	2	2	18
Chard, swiss, raw	1 cup	1	0	1	7
Chayote, chopped, boiled, drained	½ cup	4	2	2	19
Chayote, chopped, raw	1 cup	6	4	2	25
Collards, chopped, boiled, drained	½ cup	5	2	3	25
Collards, chopped, frozen, boiled, drained	½ cup	6	4	2	31
Collards, chopped, raw	1 cup	2	1	1	11
Corn, canned, w/red & green peppers	½ cup	21	21	na	85
Corn, canned, white	½ cup	20	18	2	83
Corn, canned, white, sweet, whole kernel, canned	½ cup	15	13	2	66
Corn, canned, white, sweet, whole kernel	½ cup	20	19	1	82

VEGETABLES AND VEGETABLE JUICES 351

FOOD	SERVING	TOTAL CARBS (G)	NET CARBS (G)	FIBER (G)	CALORIES
Corn, fresh, white, sweet, boiled, drained	½ cup	21	19	2	89
Corn, frozen, white, sweet, boiled, drained	½ cup	16	14	2	66
Corn, white, sweet, on the cob	1 ear	14	13	1	59
Corn, canned, yellow, sweet	½ cup	15	13	2	66
Corn, fresh, yellow, sweet, boiled, drained	½ cup	20	17	3	88
Corn on the cob, fresh, yellow, sweet, boiled, drained	1 ear	19	17	2	83
Corn cut off the cob, frozen, yellow, sweet, boiled, drained	½ cup	16	14	2	66
Corn, sweet, white or yellow, canned, cream style	½ cup	23	22	1	92
Corn pudding, home prepared	1 cup	32	32	0	272
Cucumber, peeled, raw, chopped	1 cup	3	2	1	16
Cucumber, peeled, raw, sliced	1 cup	3	2	1	14
Cucumber, peeled, raw, large (8¼" long)	1 cucumber	7	5	2	34
Cucumber, peeled, raw, medium	1 cucumber	5	4	1	24
Cucumber, peeled, raw, small (6⅜" long)	1 cucumber	4	3	1	19

VEGETABLES AND VEGETABLE JUICES

FOOD	SERVING	TOTAL CARBS (G)	NET CARBS (G)	FIBER (G)	CALORIES
Cucumber, w/peel, raw, slices	1 cup	3	2	1	14
Cucumber, w/peel, raw, large (8¼" long)	1 cucumber	8	6	2	39
Dandelion greens, chopped, boiled, drained	½ cup	3	1.5	1.5	17
Dandelion greens, raw, chopped	1 cup	5	3	2	25
Eggplant, cubed, boiled, drained	½ cup	3	2	1	14
Eggplant, raw, cubed	1 cup	5	3	2	21
Endive, raw, chopped	1 cup	2	0	2	9
Grape leaves, raw	1 cup	2	.5	1.5	13
Hubbard squash, baked, cubed	½ cup	11	11	na	51
Hubbard squash, boiled, mashed	½ cup	8	5	3	35
Jicama, raw, sliced	1 cup	11	5	6	46
Kale, chopped, boiled, drained, w/o salt	½ cup	4	3	1	18
Kale, frozen, chopped, boiled, drained	½ cup	3	2	1	20
Kale, raw, chopped	1 cup	7	6	1	34
Kale, Scotch, chopped, boiled, drained	½ cup	4	3	1	18
Kale, Scotch, raw, chopped	1 cup	6	5	1	28
Kohlrabi, sliced, boiled, drained	½ cup	6	5	1	24

VEGETABLES AND VEGETABLE JUICES

FOOD	SERVING	TOTAL CARBS (G)	NET CARBS (G)	FIBER (G)	CALORIES
Kohlrabi, raw	1 cup	8	3	5	36
Leeks (bulb & lower leaf portion), boiled, drained	1 leek	10	9	1	38
Leeks, chopped (bulb & lower leaf portion), boiled, drained	½ cup	4	3	t	16
Leeks, chopped, raw (bulb & lower leaf portion)	1 cup	13	11	2	54
Leeks, raw (bulb & lower leaf portion)	1 leek	13	11	2	54
Lettuce, shredded, raw, butterhead, Boston, & Bibb types	1 cup	1	0	1	7
Lettuce, shredded, raw, cos or romaine	1 cup	1	0	1	8
Lettuce, shredded, raw, iceberg	1 cup	1	0	1	7
Lettuce, shredded, raw, loose-leaf	1 cup	2	1	1	10
Lettuce, shredded, raw, radicchio	1 cup	2	2	t	9
Mushrooms, raw, cremini or Italian	6 pieces	4	3.5	.5	18
Mushrooms, canned, drained	½ cup	4	2	2	19
Mushrooms, boiled, drained	½ cup	4	2	2	21
Mushrooms, boiled, drained	6 pieces	4	2	2	19

354 VEGETABLES AND VEGETABLE JUICES

FOOD	SERVING	TOTAL CARBS (G)	NET CARBS (G)	FIBER (G)	CALORIES
Mushrooms, raw, enoki	6 pieces (large)	2	1	1	10
Mushrooms, raw, enoki	6 pieces (medium)	1	.5	.5	6
Mushrooms, raw, slices or pieces	1 cup	3	2	1	18
Mushrooms, raw, whole	1 cup	4	3	1	24
Mushrooms, raw	6 pieces (large)	6	4	2	35
Mushrooms, raw	6 pieces (medium)	5	4	1	27
Mushrooms, raw portobello	4 slices	4	1	3	20
Mushrooms, cooked, pieces, shiitake	½ cup	10	8.5	1.5	40
Mushrooms, cooked, whole, shiitake	6 pieces	15	13	2	59
Mushrooms, dried, shiitake	6 mushrooms	17	14	3	67
Mushrooms, canned, straw, drained	½ cup	4	2	2	29
Okra, frozen, boiled, drained	½ cup	5	2	3	26
Okra, raw	1 cup	8	5	3	33
Okra, raw	6 pods	5	3	2	24
Okra, slices, boiled, drained	½ cup	6	4	2	26
Okra, whole, boiled, drained	6 pods	5	3	2	20
Onions, boiled, drained	½ cup	11	9.5	1.5	46
Onions, boiled, drained	1 large	13	11	2	56
Onions, boiled, drained	1 medium	10	9	1	41
Onions, boiled, drained	1 small	6	5	1	26
Onions, canned	½ cup	5	4	1	21

VEGETABLES AND VEGETABLE JUICES

FOOD	SERVING	TOTAL CARBS (G)	NET CARBS (G)	FIBER (G)	CALORIES
Onions, dehydrated flakes	¼ cup	12	11	1	49
Onions, frozen, chopped, boiled, drained	½ cup	7	5	2	29
Onions, raw, chopped	1 cup	14	11	3	61
Onions, raw, sliced	1 cup	10	8	2	44
Onions, raw, slice (¼" thick)	1 slice	3	2	1	14
Onions, raw, slice (⅛" thick)	1 slice	1	1	t	5
Onions, raw, whole	1 large	13	10	3	57
Onions, raw, whole	1 medium	9	7	2	42
Onions, raw, whole	1 small	6	5	1	27
Onions, raw, chopped, spring or scallions (tops & bulbs)	1 cup	7	4	3	32
Onions, raw, whole spring or scallions (tops & bulbs)	1 large	2	1	1	8
Onions, raw, whole spring or scallions (tops & bulbs)	1 medium	1	0	t	5
Onions, raw, whole spring or scallions (tops & bulbs)	1 small	t	t	t	2
Onion rings, breaded, par fried, frozen, prepared, heated in oven	1 cup	18	17	1	195
Palm, hearts, canned	½ cup	3	1	2	20
Palm, hearts, canned	3 pieces	5	3	2	28

VEGETABLES AND VEGETABLE JUICES

FOOD	SERVING	TOTAL CARBS (G)	NET CARBS (G)	FIBER (G)	CALORIES
Parsley, freeze dried	¼ cup	t	t	.5	4
Parsley, raw	1 cup	4	2	2	22
Parsley, raw	6 sprigs	t	t	t	2
Parsnips, raw	1 cup	24	17.5	6.5	100
Parsnips, sliced, boiled, drained	½ cup	15	12	3	63
Peas & carrots, canned	½ cup	11	8	3	48
Peas, edible-podded, fresh, boiled, drained	½ cup	6	4	2	34
Peas, edible-podded, frozen, boiled, drained	½ cup	7	4.5	2.5	42
Peas, green, canned	½ cup	11	7.5	3.5	59
Peas, green, fresh, boiled, drained	½ cup	13	9	4	67
Peas, green, frozen, boiled, drained	½ cup	11	7	4	62
Peas, pigeon, fresh, boiled	½ cup	20	14	6	102
Peas & onions, canned	½ cup	5	4	1	31
Peas & onions, frozen, boiled, drained	½ cup	8	6	2	41
Peppers, chili, green, canned	½ cup	3	2	1	15
Peppers, hot chili, sun dried	6 peppers	2	1	1	10
Peppers, hot chili, green, chopped, canned, pods	½ cup	3	2	1	14

VEGETABLES AND VEGETABLE JUICES 357

FOOD	SERVING	TOTAL CARBS (G)	NET CARBS (G)	FIBER (G)	CALORIES
Peppers, hot chili, green, whole, canned	1 pepper	4	3	1	15
Peppers, hot chili, green, chopped, raw	1 cup	14	12	2	60
Peppers, hot chili, green, whole, raw	1 pepper	4	3	1	18
Peppers, chili, red, chopped, canned	½ cup	3	2	1	14
Peppers, hot chili, red, whole, canned	1 pepper	4	3	1	15
Peppers, hot chili, red, chopped, raw	1 cup	14	12	2	60
Peppers, hot chili, red, whole, raw	1 pepper	4	3	1	18
Peppers, Hungarian, raw	1 pepper	2	2	na	8
Peppers, jalapeño, chopped, canned	½ cup	3	1	2	18
Peppers, jalapeño, sliced, canned	½ cup	2	1	1	14
Peppers, jalapeño, whole, canned	1 pepper	1	0	1	6
Peppers, jalapeño, whole, raw	1 pepper	1	1	t	4
Peppers, sweet, green, halves, canned	½ cup	3	2	1	13
Peppers, sweet, green, chopped, boiled, drained	½ cup	5	4	1	19

VEGETABLES AND VEGETABLE JUICES

FOOD	SERVING	TOTAL CARBS (G)	NET CARBS (G)	FIBER (G)	CALORIES
Peppers, sweet, green, chopped, raw	1 cup	10	7	3	40
Peppers, sweet, green, slices, raw	1 cup	6	4	2	25
Peppers, sweet, green, large, raw	1 pepper	11	8	3	44
Peppers, sweet, green, medium, raw	1 pepper	8	6	2	32
Peppers, sweet, green, small, raw	1 pepper	5	4	1	20
Peppers, sweet, green, rings, raw	6 rings	4	3	1	16
Peppers, sweet, green, rings, raw	6 strips	1	1	t	4
Peppers, sweet, red, chopped, boiled, drained	½ cup	5	4	1	19
Peppers, sweet, red, chopped, raw	1 cup	10	7	3	40
Peppers, sweet, red, slices, raw	1 cup	6	4	2	25
Peppers, sweet, red, large, raw	1 pepper	11	8	3	44
Peppers, sweet, red, medium, raw	1 pepper	8	6	2	32
Peppers, sweet, red, small, raw	1 pepper	5	3.5	1.5	20
Peppers, sweet, yellow, large, raw	1 pepper	12	10	2	50
Peppers, sweet, yellow, strips, raw	6 strips	2	2	t	8

VEGETABLES AND VEGETABLE JUICES

FOOD	SERVING	TOTAL CARBS (G)	NET CARBS (G)	FIBER (G)	CALORIES
Potatoes, au gratin, home prepared from recipe using butter	1 cup	28	24	4	323
Potatoes, au gratin, home prepared from recipe using margarine	1 cup	28	24	4	323
Potatoes, au gratin, dry mix, prepared w/water, whole milk & butter	0.17 package (5.5 oz)	18	17	1	130
Potato, baked w/skin	1 medium	37	33	4	161
Potato, boiled w/o skin	1 medium	33	30	3	144
Potatoes, canned, drained	½ cup	12	10	2	54
Potatoes, french fried, frozen, home prepared, heated in oven	20 strips	31	29	3	200
Potatoes, french fried, frozen, home prepared, heated in oven	15 strips	23	21	2	150
Potatoes, french fried, frozen, pan fried, cottage cut, prepared, heated in oven	15 strips	26	24	2	164
Potatoes, hashed brown, frozen, plain, prepared	1 patty, oval (3" x 1½" x ½")	8	7	1	63
Potatoes, hashed brown, frozen, plain, prepared w/butter sauce	1 patty, oval (3" x 1½" x ½")	7	6	1	52
Potatoes, hashed brown, home prepared	1 cup	33	30	3	326

VEGETABLES AND VEGETABLE JUICES

FOOD	SERVING	TOTAL CARBS (G)	NET CARBS (G)	FIBER (G)	CALORIES
Potatoes, mashed, dehydrated, prepared from flakes w/o milk, whole milk & butter added	½ cup	16	14	2	119
Potatoes, mashed, dehydrated, prepared from granules w/milk, water & margarine added	½ cup	14	12	2	83
Potatoes, mashed, dehydrated, prepared from granules w/o milk, whole milk & butter added	½ cup	15	13	2	113
Potatoes, mashed, home prepared, whole milk added	½ cup	18	16	2	81
Potatoes, mashed, home prepared, whole milk & butter added	½ cup	18	16	2	111
Potatoes, mashed, home prepared, whole milk & margarine added	½ cup	18	16	2	111
Potatoes, O'Brien, frozen, unprepared	½ cup	17	15	2	76
Potato puffs, frozen, prepared	1 cup	39	35	4	284
Potato salad, home prepared	1 cup	28	25	3	357

VEGETABLES AND VEGETABLE JUICES 361

FOOD	SERVING	TOTAL CARBS (G)	NET CARBS (G)	FIBER (G)	CALORIES
Potatoes, scalloped, home prepared w/butter	½ cup	13	11	2	105
Potatoes, scalloped, home prepared w/margarine	½ cup	13	11	2	105
Potatoes, scalloped, dry mix, prepared w/water, whole milk & butter	0.17 package (5.5 oz)	18	16	2	130
Potato wedges, frozen	½ cup	26	24	2	123
Potatoes, microwaved w/skin	1 medium	36	33.5	2.5	156
Potatoes, red, baked w/flesh & skin	1 medium	34	31	3	154
Potatoes, russet, baked w/flesh & skin	1 medium	37	33	4	168
Potatoes, white, baked w/flesh & skin	1 medium	36	32	4	163
Pumpkin, canned	½ cup	10	6	4	42
Pumpkin, boiled, mashed	½ cup	6	5	1	25
Radishes, Oriental, sliced, boiled, drained	½ cup	3	2	1	12
Radishes, Oriental, whole, raw	1 radish	14	9	5	61
Radishes, slices, raw	1 cup	4	2	2	23
Radish, large, raw	1 radish	t	t	t	2
Radish, medium, raw	1 radish	t	t	t	1
Radishes, white icicle, slices, raw	1 cup	3	2	1	14

362 VEGETABLES AND VEGETABLE JUICES

FOOD	SERVING	TOTAL CARBS (G)	NET CARBS (G)	FIBER (G)	CALORIES
Radishes, white icicle, whole, raw	1 radish	t	t	t	2
Rhubarb, raw, diced	1 cup	6	4	2	26
Rutabagas, cubed, boiled, drained	½ cup	7	5.5	1.5	33
Rutabagas, mashed, boiled, drained	½ cup	11	9	2	47
Sauerkraut, canned	½ cup	3	1	2	13
Seaweed, kelp, raw	2 tbsp	8	7	1	34
Shallots, chopped, raw	1 tbsp	2	2	na	7
Spinach, au gratin, frozen	1 serving	11	9	2	222
Spinach, canned	½ cup	3	0	3	22
Spinach, boiled, drained	½ cup	3	1	2	21
Spinach, creamed, frozen	1 serving	9	7	2	169
Spinach, frozen, chopped or leaf, boiled, drained	½ cup	5	2	3	27
Spinach, raw	1 cup	1	0	1	7
Spinach souffle, home prepared	1 cup	3	3	0	219
Sprouts, alfalfa, raw	1 cup	1	0	1	10
Sprouts, mung, boiled, drained	½ cup	2.5	2.5	na	13
Sprouts, mung, raw	1 cup	6	6	na	30
Squash, spaghetti, boiled or baked, drained	½ cup	5	4	1	21

VEGETABLES AND VEGETABLE JUICES

FOOD	SERVING	TOTAL CARBS (G)	NET CARBS (G)	FIBER (G)	CALORIES
Stir fry vegetables w/white rice & Oriental soy sauce, frozen	1 cup	27	25	2	130
Succotash (corn & limas), boiled, drained	½ cup	23	19	4	110
Succotash (corn & limas), canned, w/cream style corn	½ cup	23	19	4	102
Succotash (corn & limas), frozen, boiled, drained	½ cup	17	13.5	3.5	79
Summer squash, all varieties, sliced, boiled, drained	½ cup	4	3	1	18
Summer squash, all varieties, sliced, raw	1 cup	5	3	2	23
Summer squash, crookneck & straightneck, diced, canned	½ cup	3	1.5	1.5	14
Summer squash, crookneck & straightneck, mashed, canned	½ cup	4	2	2	16
Summer squash, crookneck & straightneck, slices, canned	½ cup	3	1.5	1.5	14

VEGETABLES AND VEGETABLE JUICES

FOOD	SERVING	TOTAL CARBS (G)	NET CARBS (G)	FIBER (G)	CALORIES
Summer squash, crookneck & straightneck, frozen	½ cup	5	4	1	24
Summer squash, crookneck & straightneck, slices, raw	1 cup	5	2.5	2.5	25
Sweet potato, baked in skin	½ cup	24	21	3	103
Sweet potato, baked in skin	1 medium	28	25	3	117
Sweet potato, candied, home prepared	1 potato (2½" x 2" dia)	29	26	3	144
Sweet potato, canned, syrup pack, drained solids	½ cup	25	22	3	106
Sweet potato, canned, syrup pack, w/solids & liquids	½ cup	24	21	3	101
Sweet potato, canned, mashed	½ cup	30	28	2	129
Sweet potatoes, frozen, cubes, baked	½ cup	21	19	2	88
Taro shoots, slices, cooked	½ cup	2	2	na	10
Taro shoots, slices, raw	1 cup	2	2	na	9
Tomatillos, medium, raw	1 tomatillo	2	1	1	11
Tomatillos, chopped, raw	1 cup	8	5.5	2.5	42

VEGETABLES AND VEGETABLE JUICES 365

FOOD	SERVING	TOTAL CARBS (G)	NET CARBS (G)	FIBER (G)	CALORIES
Tomatoes, crushed, canned	½ cup	9	7	2	39
Tomatoes, green, chopped, raw	1 cup	9	7	2	43
Tomatoes, green, slices or wedges, raw	1 piece	1	1	t	5
Tomatoes, green, whole, raw	1 large tomato	9	7	2	44
Tomatoes, green, whole, raw	1 medium, tomato	6	5	1	30
Tomatoes, green, whole, small, raw	1 small tomato	5	4	1	22
Tomatoes, orange, chopped, raw	1 cup	5	4	1	25
Tomatoes, orange, raw	1 tomato	4	3	1	18
Tomatoes, red, canned, stewed	½ cup	9	8	1	36
Tomatoes, red, canned, wedges in tomato juice	½ cup	8	8	na	34
Tomatoes, red, whole, canned	½ cup	5	4	1	23
Tomatoes, red, canned, w/green chiles	½ cup	4	4	na	18
Tomatoes, red, boiled	½ cup	7	6	1	32
Tomatoes, red, slices (¼" thick)	1 slice	1	1	t	4
Tomatoes, red (¼ of a medium tomato), raw	1 wedge	1	1	t	7
Tomatoes, red, whole, boiled	2 medium tomatoes	14	11.5	2.5	66

VEGETABLES AND VEGETABLE JUICES

FOOD	SERVING	TOTAL CARBS (G)	NET CARBS (G)	FIBER (G)	CALORIES
Tomatoes, red, whole, raw	1 large tomato	8	6	2	38
Tomatoes, red, whole, raw	1 medium tomato	6	5	1	26
Tomatoes, red, whole, raw	1 small tomato	4	3	1	19
Tomatoes, red, stewed	½ cup	7	6	1	40
Tomatoes, cherry, raw	1 cup	7	5	2	31
Tomatoes, cherry, raw	1 tomato	1	1	t	4
Tomatoes, red, chopped, raw	1 cup	8	6	2	38
Tomatoes, roma (Italian), raw	1 tomato	3	2	1	13
Tomatoes, sun dried	½ cup	15	12	3	70
Tomatoes, sun dried, packed in oil, drained	1 cup	26	20	6	234
Tomatoes, sun dried	1 piece	1	1	t	5
Tomatoes, yellow, chopped, raw	1 cup	4	3	1	21
Tomatoes, yellow, whole, raw	1 tomato	6	4.5	1.5	32
Tomato paste	¼ cup	12	9.5	2.5	53
Tomato puree	½ cup	12	9.5	2.5	50
Tomato sauce, canned	½ cup	9	7	2	37
Tomato sauce, canned, Spanish style	½ cup	9	7	2	40
Tomato sauce, canned, w/mushrooms	½ cup	10	8	2	43
Tomato sauce, canned, w/onions	½ cup	12	10	2	51

VEGETABLES AND VEGETABLE JUICES

FOOD	SERVING	TOTAL CARBS (G)	NET CARBS (G)	FIBER (G)	CALORIES
Tomato sauce, canned, w/onions, green peppers & celery	½ cup	11	9	2	51
Tomato sauce, canned, w/tomato tidbits	½ cup	9	7	2	39
Turnips, cubes, boiled, drained	½ cup	4	2	2	16
Turnips, mashed, boiled, drained	½ cup	6	4	2	24
Turnips, frozen, boiled, drained	½ cup	3	1	2	18
Turnip greens & turnips, frozen, boiled, drained	½ cup	2	.5	1.5	15
Vegetables, mixed, canned	½ cup	8	6	2	38
Vegetables, mixed, frozen, boiled, drained	½ cup	12	8	4	54
Water chestnuts, Chinese, slices, canned	½ cup	9	7	2	35
Watercress, chopped, raw	1 cup	t	t	t	4
Watercress, raw	10 sprigs	t	t	t	3
Winter squash, all varieties, baked	½ cup	9	6	3	40
Zucchini, frozen, boiled, drained	½ cup	4	3	1	19
Zucchini, sliced, boiled, drained	½ cup	4	3	1	14

YOGURT

FOOD	SERVING	TOTAL CARBS (G)	NET CARBS (G)	FIBER (G)	CALORIES
Zucchini, mashed, boiled, drained	½ cup	5	3	2	19
Zucchini, chopped, raw	1 cup	4	2.5	1.5	17
VEGETABLE JUICES					
Carrot juice, canned	1 cup	22	20	2	94
Clam & tomato juice	1 can (5.5 oz)	18	18	t	80
Mixed vegetable & fruit juice drink	1 serving	28	27	t	110
Tomato juice	1 cup	10	9	1	41
Vegetable juice cocktail, canned	1 cup	11	9	2	46
YOGURT					
Frozen yogurt, hard, low fat, all flavors	½ cup	26	26	0	na
Frozen yogurt, nonfat, w/low-calorie sweetener	½ cup	18	16	2	100
Frozen yogurt, chocolate, soft serve	½ cup	18	16	2	71
Frozen yogurt, vanilla, soft serve	½ cup	17	17	0	63
Fruit flavored, creamy style, low fat (1% milkfat)	1 cup	45	44	1	125
Fruit flavored, low fat (1% milkfat)	1 small container (4.4 oz)	27	27	t	56
Fruit flavored, low fat (1% milkfat)	1 cup	41	40.5	.5	118
Fruit flavored, whole fat	1 cup	38	38	0	156
Light Yogurt (Yoplait)	6 oz	19	19	0	100

FOOD	SERVING	TOTAL CARBS (G)	NET CARBS (G)	FIBER (G)	CALORIES
Light 'n Fit Carb Control Peaches 'n Cream (Dannon)	4 oz	3	3	0	60
Light 'n Fit Carb Control Raspberries 'n Cream (Dannon)	4 oz	3	3	0	60
Light 'n Fit Carb Control Strawberry 'n Cream (Dannon)	4 oz	3	3	0	60
Light 'n Fit Carb Control Vanilla Cream (Dannon)	4 oz	3	3	0	60
Nonfat, no-sugar yogurt, vanilla, lemon, maple or coffee flavor	1 cup	18	18	0	105
Nonfat yogurt, strawberry, w/ aspartame & fructose (Kraft Breyers Light)	1 cup	22	22	0	125
Plain yogurt, low fat	1 cup	16	16	0	143
Plain yogurt, skim milk	1 cup	17	17	0	127
Plain yogurt, whole milk	1 cup	11	11	0	139
Reduced Sugar, Lowfat Yogurt, Blueberry (Hood, Carb Countdown)	1 container (6 oz)	4	3	0	80
Reduced Sugar, Lowfat Yogurt, Peach (Hood, Carb Countdown)	1 container (6 oz)	4	3	0	80

YOGURT

FOOD	SERVING	TOTAL CARBS (G)	NET CARBS (G)	FIBER (G)	CALORIES
Reduced Sugar, Lowfat Yogurt, Strawberry Banana (Hood, Carb Countdown)	1 container (6 oz)	4	3	0	80
Reduced Sugar, Lowfat Yogurt, Strawberry (Hood, Carb Countdown)	1 container (6 oz)	4	3	0	80
Reduced Sugar, Lowfat Yogurt, French Vanilla (Hood, Carb Countdown)	1 container (6 oz)	4	3	0	80
Yogurt fruit smoothies, bottled	1 bottle (10 fl oz)	52	52	0	130
Yogurt Smoothies, Black Cherry, Bottled (Hood, Carb Countdown)	1 bottle (10 oz)	4	3	0	100
Yogurt Smoothies, Peach, Bottled (Hood, Carb Countdown)	1 bottle (10 oz)	4	3	0	100
Yogurt Smoothies, Strawberry Banana, Bottled (Hood, Carb Countdown)	1 bottle (10 oz)	4	3	0	100
Yogurt Smoothies, Strawberry, Bottled (Hood, Carb Countdown)	1 bottle (10 oz)	4	3	0	100

APPENDIX: LOW-CARB FOOD SOURCES

Many of the low-carb foods listed in *The Essential Net Carb Counter* can be purchased online from the following websites:

a la Carb—The Low Carb & Sugar Free Menu	www.alacarb.com
Atkins Diet & Low Carbohydrate Weight-Loss Support	www.lowcarb.ca
Synergy Diet	www.synergydiet.com
Atkins	www.atkins.com
Low Carb Nexus	www.lowcarbnexus.com
Keto Foods	www.ketofoods.com
Russell Stover	www.russellstover.com
Fantastic Foods	www.fantasticfoods.com
Hood, Carb Countdown	www.hphood.com

Not sure what to read next?

Visit Pocket Books online at
www.simonsays.com

Reading suggestions for
you and your reading group
New release news
Author appearances
Online chats with your favorite writers
Special offers
Order books online
And much, much more!

POCKET BOOKS
A Division of Simon & Schuster
A CBS COMPANY

POCKET STAR BOOKS
A Division of Simon & Schuster
A CBS COMPANY

13456

Printed in Great Britain
by Amazon.co.uk, Ltd.,
Marston Gate.